World Culture and Digestion

Unlocking Natural Gut Health Through Global Diets

D.R. Darcy

Table of Contents

The Gut:

Nourishing the Core for Optimal Wellness

Everyday we live, and every meal we eat influences the great microbial organ inside us–for better or for worse. –Guilia Enders

Explore the vital connection between your gut and overall health. Beyond digestion, the gut impacts immunity and well-being. Discover its intricacies and the power of nutrition for holistic wellness. Gain critical insights to effectively nourish the gut and enhance your health.

The Importance of Gut Health for Overall Well-Being

Gut health is pivotal in maintaining overall well-being and vitality. The gastrointestinal tract, often called the gut, is home to countless bacteria types that form a complex ecosystem known as the gut microbiota. These microscopic inhabitants influence numerous aspects of our health, from digestion and nutrient absorption to immune function and mental well-being.

One of the primary functions of a healthy gut is efficient digestion and nutrient absorption. The gut digests food into smaller particles and absorbs essential nutrients such as vitamins, minerals, and amino acids. A well-functioning gut ensures that these nutrients are appropriately assimilated into the bloodstream, providing the body with the fuel it needs to thrive. Conversely, poor gut health can lead to nutrient deficiencies, impacting energy levels, immune function, and overall vitality.

Another crucial aspect of gut health is its influence on the immune system. The gut plays home to a large portion of our immune cells, and a balanced gut microbiota helps regulate immune responses. A healthy gut microbiota strengthens the intestinal barrier, preventing unhealthy pathogens from entering the bloodstream and triggering immune responses. Furthermore, beneficial gut bacteria produce compounds that support immune function and suppress the growth of harmful microorganisms. By promoting a robust immune system, a healthy gut can help defend against infections, allergies, and autoimmune conditions.

Emerging research also highlights the gut-brain connection, demonstrating the significant impact of gut health on mental well-being. The brain and the gut liaise bidirectionally through various pathways, such as the vagus nerve and the production of neurotransmitters. Studies have linked an imbalance in gut bacteria to conditions like anxiety, depression, and even neurodegenerative disorders (Clapp et al., 2017). Therefore, nurturing a diverse and thriving gut microbiota is essential for maintaining optimal mental health.

Governing gut health requires a multifaceted approach. A well-rounded diet rich in fiber, fruits, vegetables, and fermented foods promotes the growth of beneficial gut bacteria. Physical activity supports healthy gut motility and enhances microbial diversity. Minimizing stress levels and getting sufficient sleep also contribute to a healthy gut.

By prioritizing gut health through proper nutrition, exercise, and stress management, we can unlock the full potential of our bodies and lead vibrant, healthy lives.

Caring for Ingested Food for Optimal Function

Did you know that approximately 70-80% of our immune system is located in the gut? (Cohen, 2021).

Taking care of ingested food is essential for optimal function because of the reasons mentioned below.

Gut Health: Our gut health is crucial for overall well-being. Nurturing a diverse and balanced gut microbiota through mindful food choices promotes optimal gut health.

Energy Levels and Performance: The quality of the food we consume affects our energy levels and overall performance. Highly processed foods lacking in essential nutrients can lead to energy crashes and sluggishness. Conversely, a diet rich in whole foods, including fruits, vegetables, lean proteins, and whole grains, supplies sustained energy and supports optimal cognitive and physical function.

Disease Prevention: Poor dietary habits have been linked to various chronic diseases, including type 2 diabetes, obesity, heart disease, and certain cancers. Taking care of the ingested food by making healthier choices lowers the risk of developing these conditions and promotes long-term health.

The Gut and its Function–A Brief Overview

The gut, also named the gastrointestinal tract, is an intricate system that plays a crucial role in various physiological processes. From digestion and nutrient absorption to immune function and hormone regulation, the gut performs a range of vital functions.

Here is a glance at the numerous functions of the gut:

Digestion

- The gut is in charge of dissolving food into smaller particles through mechanical and chemical processes.
- Digestive enzymes and stomach acids aid in the breakdown of proteins, fats, and carbohydrates.
- The process of peristalsis, rhythmic muscular contractions, moves food through the digestive system.

Nutrient Absorption

- The lining of the small intestine contains microscopic finger-like ridges called *villi*, which increase the surface area for nutrient absorption.
- Nutrients, including minerals, vitamins, and amino acids, are soaked up into the bloodstream and transported to cells throughout the body.

Gut Microbiota

- These gut microbiota help break down dietary fibers, produce a range of vitamins (such as vitamins B and K), and aid in digesting certain substances.

Immune Function

- A significant portion of the body's immune cells are found in the gut-associated lymphoid tissue (GALT).
- The gut acts as a barrier, preventing harmful pathogens from entering the bloodstream.
- Beneficial gut bacteria help train and modulate the immune system, promoting a healthy immune response.

Hormone Regulation

- The gut produces several hormones that regulate appetite, satiety, and digestion.
- Hormones like ghrelin, produced in the stomach, stimulate hunger, while peptides YY and leptin signal feelings of fullness.
- Gut hormones also communicate with the brain, influencing mood, stress response, and overall well-being.

Waste Elimination

- The colon, or large intestine, absorbs water and electrolytes from undigested food.
- It also acts in the primary role of eliminating waste materials in the form of feces.

The Gut's Relationship With Different Food Cultures

The gut's relationship with different food cultures is a fascinating and diverse subject. Across the globe, various cultures have distinct culinary traditions and dietary patterns that significantly impact gut health and overall well-being. Here is a concise exploration of the gut's relationship with different food cultures:

Mediterranean Diet

The Mediterranean diet, prevalent in countries like Greece, Italy, and Spain, emphasizes fresh fruits, whole grains, vegetables, legumes, nuts, and healthy fats like olive oil. This plant-centric diet is rich in fiber, antioxidants, and polyphenols, which promote diverse and beneficial gut microbiota. Studies have linked the Mediterranean diet to a decreased risk of heart disease, obesity, and certain cancers, highlighting the positive impact on gut health (Widmar et al., 2015).

Japanese Cuisine

Japanese cuisine, characterized by its emphasis on seafood, fermented foods like *miso* (a fermented paste), *natto* (fermented soybeans), and vegetables, contributes to a gut-friendly diet. Fermented foods, in particular, such as *kimchi* (a Korean dish with varied ingredients) and *tempeh* (a dish made from beans and grains), introduce beneficial bacteria to the gut and support digestion. Additionally, the Japanese diet is low in saturated fats and processed foods, promoting a healthy gut environment and reducing the risk of digestive disorders.

Indian Cuisine

Indian cuisine is known for its vibrant spices like turmeric, ginger, and cumin. These aromatics not only add flavor but also provide numerous health benefits. Turmeric, for instance, contains *curcumin*, a compound with anti-inflammatory properties that may support gut health. Consuming legumes, lentils, and fiber-rich vegetables like *okra* and spinach in Indian cuisine also contributes to a diverse gut microbiota and aids digestion.

Latin American Cuisine

Latin American cuisine varies across regions but often includes staples like beans, corn, avocados, and chili peppers. These foods are jam-packed with fiber, vitamins, and minerals, providing prebiotics that nourish beneficial gut bacteria. Additionally, including fermented foods like sauerkraut (Germany's variation for *curtido*) and traditional beverages like *chicha* (fermented alcoholic or non-alcoholic maize drink) in Latin American cultures introduce probiotics that support gut health and strengthen the immune system.

Traditional African Diets

Traditional African diets emphasize whole grains, legumes, lean proteins, and diverse vegetables. These dietary patterns contribute to high fiber intake, promoting healthy digestion and balanced gut microbiota. Fermented foods like *ogi* (fermented cereal pudding) and *kenkey* (sourdough dumplings), common in African cultures, also play a role in maintaining gut health by introducing beneficial bacteria.

The Gut's Role in Nutrient Absorption and Immune Function

The gut plays a vital role in both nutrient absorption and immune function, highlighting its significance for overall health and well-being.

Nutrient Absorption: The finger-like structures, called the *villi,* are responsible for expanding the surface section for our bodies to absorb nutrients. As food proceeds through the digestive system, it undergoes breakdown by digestive enzymes and stomach acids. The resulting smaller molecules, such as amino acids, sugars, and fatty acids, are absorbed into the bloodstream through these finger-like projections. This process ensures that essential nutrients from the ingested food, including vitamins, minerals, and macronutrients, are effectively absorbed and transported to cells throughout the body. The gut's ability to efficiently absorb and assimilate these nutrients is critical for providing the body with the building blocks and energy it needs to function optimally.

Immune Function: The gut is closely intertwined with the immune system, residing in the GALT. The gut acts as a physical barrier, preventing unhealthy pathogens and toxins from entering the bloodstream. It also houses the gut microbiota, contributing to immune regulation and defense against pathogens. The gut microbiota helps train and modulate the immune system, promoting appropriate responses to foreign invaders while preventing inappropriate immune reactions. Moreover, beneficial gut bacteria produce antimicrobial compounds and help govern the integrity of the intestinal barrier, further enhancing immune function. By supporting healthy gut microbiota through a balanced and diverse diet, we can foster optimal immune function and reduce the risk of infections, allergies, and autoimmune diseases.

The intricate relationship between nutrient absorption and immune function in the gut highlights the interconnectedness of these processes and their impact on overall health. A healthy gut environment, characterized by diverse gut microbiota and proper nutrient absorption, ensures the body receives the required nutrients for optimal functioning while supporting a robust immune system. Conversely, imbalances in the gut microbiota, inflammation, or compromised gut integrity can impair nutrient absorption and weaken immune responses. Therefore, maintaining a healthy gut through a balanced diet, regular physical activity, stress management, and adequate sleep are essential for promoting optimal nutrient absorption and immune function. By nurturing our gut health, we support the foundation for overall well-being and resilience against diseases and infections.

That said, let us take a deep dive into the all-important job of the gut in our anatomy and its various functions.

Chapter 1:

Anatomy and Functions

If there's one thing to know about the human body, it's this: the human body has a ringmaster. This ringmaster controls your digestion, your immunity, your brain, your weight, your health, and even your happiness. This ringmaster is the gut. –Nancy Mure

Unveil the marvel of the human body's intricate anatomy and digestive functions. Explore its complex systems and structures that ensure our well-being. This journey fosters an appreciation for our body's capabilities and informs health and lifestyle decisions.

The Role of the Gut in the Digestive System

The gut is a vital hub in the digestive system, breaking down and absorbing nutrients from food. It is composed of organs like the stomach, small intestine, and large intestine, working together to facilitate digestion and nutrient absorption. This process extracts essential components for maintaining health and well-being.

What Is the Digestive System?

The digestive system is a complex grid of cells, organs, and tissue components that combine to dissolve food into smaller molecules that the body can absorb and utilize.

It begins with ingesting food through the mouth and continues through the esophagus, stomach, small intestine, large intestine, and rectum, and ends with eliminating waste through the anus.

The process of digestion involves both mechanical and chemical processes.

Mechanical Digestion: This starts in the mouth with chewing and continues in the stomach and small intestine through muscle contractions that mix and propel food.

Chemical Digestion: This phase involves the action of enzymes and other substances that break down complex molecules into menial forms that can be absorbed.

Throughout the digestive system, nutrients such as carbohydrates, proteins, and fats are broken down and absorbed into the bloodstream. The liver and pancreas produce digestive juices that help break down and absorb nutrients. The small intestine is primarily responsible for the absorption of nutrients, while the large intestine absorbs water and electrolytes and helps form and eliminate waste products.

What Does the Digestive System Do?

The digestive system is vital in providing the body with key nutrients and energy for growth, repair, and maintenance. It is also closely linked to other bodily systems, such as the circulatory and endocrine systems, to ensure proper coordination and regulation of digestion and nutrient absorption.

In addition to its primary function of digestion and nutrient absorption, the digestive system also plays a vital role in the immune system. The gut hosts a vast village of beneficial gut microbiota. These bacteria aid in digesting certain dietary components, produce essential vitamins, and help protect against harmful pathogens.

Furthermore, the digestive system produces and releases hormones that regulate various bodily processes. For example, the small intestine releases hormones that control hunger and satiety, while the pancreas secretes insulin to regulate blood sugar levels.

The digestive system also acts as a barrier, preventing harmful substances from entering the bloodstream. The gut lining has a protective layer that selectively absorbs nutrients while blocking the absorption of toxins and pathogens.

Moreover, the digestive system influences overall health and well-being beyond digestion. Emerging research suggests that the gut microbiota may impact mental health and immune function and even play a part in conditions such as obesity and diabetes (Clemente et al., 2012).

Now that we know there is a relationship between gut health and our digestive systems, let us take a tour of how exactly they are related.

The Marriage Between the Gut and the Digestive System

Gut health and the digestive system share an intimate relationship, each influencing and affecting the other. When you nurture your gut health, your digestive system responds in kind, setting up a positive feedback loop of wellness.

Imagine your gut as a bustling city, teeming with diverse inhabitants. These microscopic residents help break down food, synthesize vital nutrients, and protect against harmful pathogens. Essentially, they act as dedicated workers maintaining the smooth operation of the city—the digestive system.

The food you consume acts like supplies to the city. A diet rich in diverse, high-fiber foods like fruits, vegetables, and whole grains offers a broad spectrum of nutrients, promoting a varied and balanced gut microbiota. In turn, this vibrant microbial community supports optimal digestion, converting the food into nutrients and energy more effectively.

Conversely, a poor diet can disrupt this equilibrium. Eating large quantities of processed food and sugar might appeal to less beneficial bacteria, fostering their growth. A shift in this delicate balance can lead to dysbiosis, a state of microbial imbalance, and potentially disrupt the digestive process.

Further, dysbiosis can cause inflammation, slowing down digestion and potentially leading to digestive disorders like irritable bowel syndrome (IBS), inflammatory bowel disease (IBD), and gastroesophageal reflux disease (GERD). In contrast, a healthy gut microbiota can help control inflammation, ensuring your digestive system stays robust and resilient.

Probiotics, often called "good bacteria," can also contribute to this beneficial relationship. Found in fermented foods like kefir, nato, and sourdough bread or taken as supplements, probiotics can replenish and diversify the gut microbiota, improving digestion and nutrient absorption.

Another essential factor that bridges gut health and the digestive system is gut motility—the movement of the muscles in the gastrointestinal tract. Imbalances in the gut microbiota can affect gut motility, leading to conditions like constipation or diarrhea. However, maintaining a healthy microbiota can promote regular and balanced gut motility, ensuring the digestive system functions smoothly.

In essence, taking care of gut health involves nurturing a thriving, diverse gut microbiota, and the rewards for doing so include optimal digestion and minimized risk of digestive disorders. So, think of your dietary choices as direct messages to the city workers in the gut. When you send the right supplies, you help them keep your city—the digestive system—running smoothly.

But what are the different components of the gut and their respective roles in our digestive systems?

The Different Gut Components and Their Digestive Functions

The gut, often known as the digestive system, acts as the body's nutritional powerhouse, transforming food into energy and nutrients. This intricate system comprises several organs, each with distinct responsibilities.

Mouth

Starting the journey is the mouth. Not only does it welcome food into your body, but it also initiates the digestion process. Chewing breaks food into smaller pieces, while salivary enzymes break down complex carbohydrates into simpler sugars.

Esophagus

Next up, the esophagus acts like a transport tunnel. Through the rhythmic muscle contractions of peristalsis, it safely delivers food from the mouth to the stomach.

Stomach

Entering the stomach, you find a muscular sac that churns food into a liquid mixture known as chyme. Gastric juice, a potent mix of hydrochloric acid and enzymes, breaks down proteins, while mucus protects the stomach lining from the acid.

Small Intestine

Beyond the stomach, the small intestine comes into play. This long, twisting tube is a hotbed for nutrient absorption. With the help of bile from the liver and gallbladder, it emulsifies fats, making them easier for the body to absorb. Meanwhile, pancreatic enzymes break down carbohydrates, proteins, and fats. The small intestine's lining, dotted with millions of tiny villi and microvilli, soaks up nutrients and shuttles them into the bloodstream.

Large Intestine

Next in the digestive journey is the colon (large intestine). Though most digestion and absorption occur before the chyme reaches the colon, it still plays a crucial role. The colon absorbs the remaining water, electrolytes, and some vitamins produced by gut bacteria. It also compacts waste into feces.

Rectum

This is the terminal section of the large intestine, which is a temporary storage area for feces.

Anus

Finally, the anus is the exit point of the digestive system, releasing waste from the body.

Moreover, the liver, pancreas, and gallbladder are essential for digestion, although not technically part of the gut. The liver produces bile to help digest fats, the pancreas secretes digestive enzymes, and the gallbladder stores and releases bile into the small intestine.

From the mouth to the anus, with several essential stops in between, each part has a vital role to play. Maintaining a healthy gut is, therefore, crucial for overall health and wellness.

Ok, great, you may ask, but how does it impact my overall health exactly?

Gut Microbiota and How It Impacts Overall Health

The gut microbiota resides in the gut, primarily in the colon. They are not merely passive inhabitants, but active players in our health. So let us delve into how they influence well-being beyond digestion.

Firstly, our gut microbiota has a prominent role in nutrient synthesis. Certain gut bacteria can produce vitamins, like vitamin K and some B vitamins, essential for various bodily functions. For example, B vitamins help the body convert food into energy, while vitamin K plays a crucial role in blood clotting.

Moreover, gut bacteria can break down dietary fiber—indigestible plant material—that your body cannot digest. During this process, the gut microbiota create components such as propionate, butyrate, and acetate, otherwise known as short-chain fatty acids (SCFAs). These SCFAs nourish the gut lining, potentially reducing the risk of inflammatory diseases like Crohn's disease and ulcerative colitis.

Another area where gut microbiota exert influence is the immune system. It teaches your immune cells to differentiate between friendly and harmful invaders, fostering immune tolerance. A balanced gut microbiota helps prepare the immune system for threats while avoiding unnecessary attacks on harmless bacteria.

Gut microbiota can also impact brain health, thanks to the gut-brain axis—a communication channel between our gut and brain. For instance, some gut bacteria can produce neurotransmitters, like serotonin and dopamine, influencing mood and behavior. A healthy gut microbiota could thus support mental well-being and potentially help manage conditions like anxiety and depression.

Interestingly, research also suggests links between gut microbiota and metabolic health. Dysbiosis, or microbial imbalance, might contribute to metabolic disorders like obesity and type 2 diabetes (Kim et al., 2020). Conversely, diverse gut microbiota could help maintain a healthy weight and glucose metabolism.

An example of this link is the case of *Akkermansia muciniphila*—a gut bacterium associated with healthy metabolic status. Some studies suggest that people with a higher abundance of A. muciniphila might have a lower risk of developing obesity and diabetes (Rodrigues et al., 2022).

Finally, gut microbiota might influence heart health. Certain gut bacteria can convert dietary l-carnitine and choline—found in red meat and eggs—into trimethylamine, which the liver converts into trimethylamine N-oxide (TMAO). High TMAO levels are linked to an increased risk of cardiovascular diseases.

So, it is clear—the gut microbiota wears many hats. From synthesizing nutrients to training our immune system, shaping brain health, influencing metabolic wellness, and potentially affecting heart health, it has far-reaching impacts on our overall well-being. Thus, nourishing a diverse and balanced gut microbiota should be a priority in our health journey.

Next up, we explore the connection between the brain and the gut.

The Gut-Brain Connection

The gut-brain axis forms a complex communication network critical for maintaining health and well-being. This axis incorporates the central nervous system, the gut microbiota, the enteric nervous system (often called the "second brain" in your gut), and various biochemical signaling pathways.

Allow me to break down this two-way communication system.

On one end, your brain sends signals to the gut through nerves like the vagus nerve and hormones. For example, when you are stressed, your brain triggers the release of stress hormones that can alter gut function, potentially leading to issues like stomach upset or changes in appetite.

On the other end, your gut communicates with the brain. One way is via the enteric nervous system, which can operate independently but also communicates with the central nervous system. However, your gut microbiota also plays a significant role in this dialogue.

Certain gut bacteria can produce neurotransmitters—chemical messengers that transmit signals in the brain. For instance, a substantial portion of the body's serotonin, a neurotransmitter crucial for mood regulation, is produced in your gut. Changes in gut microbiota may impact serotonin production, potentially influencing mood and overall mental health.

Consider this everyday scenario. Do you know that "butterflies in your stomach" feeling before a big presentation or a stressful event? This is the gut responding to your brain's stress signals. In response, the gut might slow down or speed up digestion, leading to discomfort or an "unsettled" feeling.

Moreover, an imbalance in the gut microbiota might contribute to mental health conditions. For instance, research suggests a potential link between gut microbiota and conditions like depression and anxiety (Kumar et al., 2023). Conversely, a balanced and diverse gut microbiota might support better mental health (Altas Biomed, 2020).

Even our memory and cognitive function might be influenced by our gut health. For instance, gut microbiota can affect the production of other neurotransmitters, like dopamine and glutamate, which are vital for learning and memory.

The gut-brain axis can also influence our eating behaviors and taste preferences. For instance, our gut microbiota might signal the brain to crave foods they can thrive on—whether fruits and vegetables or sugary, fatty foods.

In summary, the gut and brain share a deep connection that influences various aspects of our health—from digestion and mood to cognitive function and food cravings. The complex dialogue between the gut and brain underpins why taking care of your gut health could also mean taking care of your brain health. The gut-brain axis is yet another fascinating example of how interconnected the human body truly is.

We conclude this chapter by discovering how mood and appetite are influenced by good gut health.

The Influence of the Connection on Mood and Appetite

The intricate link between gut health, mood, and appetite presents an exciting frontier in health research. Unpacking this connection can help us understand how the foods we eat might affect our feelings and desires for different types of food.

Mood

First, let us examine how gut health can influence mood. The gut-brain axis is critical here. Certain gut bacteria can produce neurotransmitters like serotonin, often called the "feel-good" hormone, which plays a vital role in mood regulation.

For instance, consider the day you ate a greasy, fast-food meal. You might have felt sluggish or irritable afterward. This could be because such a meal, lacking in fiber and rich in fats, might not support the development of beneficial gut bacteria, which can produce mood-regulating neurotransmitters.

Furthermore, gut bacteria can generate other bioactive molecules that can cross the blood-brain barrier and potentially influence brain function and mood. Thus, a balanced gut microbiota could contribute to better mood regulation, whereas an imbalanced one could possibly contribute to mood disorders.

Appetite

Now, let us move on to appetite. Our gut microbiota can affect our desire to consume what we crave, and how much we eat. Some gut bacteria can break down dietary fiber into SCFAs, stimulating the release of appetite-regulating hormones. For example, SCFAs can promote the secretion of peptides like GLP-1 and PYY, which help us feel full and satisfied after eating.

Remember when you could not resist a second slice of cake, even though you were full? This might be because a diet high in sugar can foster the growth of certain gut bacteria that benefit from such foods, which could influence the brain to crave more sugary treats.

However, the influence of gut microbiota on appetite is not always negative. For instance, a diverse gut microbiota, fostered by a varied, fiber-rich diet, might promote the production of

SCFAs and appetite-regulating hormones, helping us feel satisfied and curb unnecessary snacking.

In essence, while the connection between gut health, mood, and appetite is complex, it underscores the potential power of dietary choices. A balanced and diverse gut microbiota could support better mood regulation and healthier eating behaviors, offering a compelling reason to nourish our gut microbiota through a varied, fiber-rich diet.

Conversely, an imbalanced gut microbiota might contribute to mood disturbances and unhealthy eating behaviors, underscoring the potential downside of neglecting gut health (Terry et al., 2022).

In the next chapter, you can look forward to the next destination in our journey about food and cultural diversity.

Chapter 2:

Cultural Diversity in Food

Food is a central activity of mankind and one of the single most significant trademarks of a culture. –Mark Kurlansky

Cultural diversity brings a delicious array of foods and culinary practices to the global table. From the North African folk drinking apple cider vinegar to fiber-rich lentils in Indian cuisine, these diverse foods shape our taste experiences and our gut health. A diet that embraces a variety of culturally diverse foods can foster robust, varied gut microbiota, contributing to better digestive and overall health.

Conversely, a less varied diet, typical of highly processed Western diets, might result in less diverse gut microbiota, potentially impacting health negatively (Singh et al., 2017).

Let us explore how the world's pantry influences our gut health and wellness.

Examples of Various Global Food Cultures

Global food cultures offer a delightful mosaic of flavors, ingredients, and cooking techniques. They not only reflect the diversity of the world's cultures, but they also influence our health in unique ways.

Let us embark on a culinary journey around the globe.

Asia

Japanese cuisine is a prime example of a diet that promotes gut health. It is rich in fermented foods like *katsuobushi* (dried bonito) and *tsukemono* (pickles), which introduce beneficial bacteria to our gut microbiota. Also, Japanese people traditionally consume various fresh, minimally processed foods, such as fish and vegetables. The downside? Some traditional Japanese dishes are high in salt, which can impact cardiovascular health if consumed excessively.

The Mediterranean Belt

Heading west, we arrive in the Mediterranean region. The Mediterranean diet, encompassing Greek (*dolmades*), Italian (minestrone), Spanish (Andalusian *Gazpacho*), and other regional cuisines, is globally recognized for its health benefits. It is rich in whole grains, fruits, vegetables, olive oil, and lean proteins like fish. These foods supply diverse nutrients and fiber, fostering healthy gut microbiota. However, remember that while the Mediterranean diet promotes moderate wine consumption, excessive alcohol can have negative health impacts.

Mexico

Crossing the Atlantic, let us explore traditional Mexican cuisine. We can find healthy food in dishes such as baked corn tortillas. Mexican food, a UNESCO-designated cultural heritage, boasts rich flavors and diverse ingredients, including beans, corn, tomatoes, and a variety of chilies. Beans, a prebiotic food, feed the beneficial bacteria in the gut, promoting healthy microbiota. One potential con is the high calorie and fat content in some popular dishes, which could contribute to obesity if overconsumed.

East Africa

Next, consider the traditional diet of the Maasai, a group in East Africa. Their diet consists mainly of honey, meat, milk, and tree bark. While this might seem unusual to many, it has sustained them for centuries. However, the limited variety of foods could potentially result in a less diverse gut microbiota and may lack certain nutrients.

India

In India, a myriad of regional cuisines offers a rich selection of dishes such as *kitchari* (dal and basmati rice), *tikka masala* (roasted marinated chicken cubes), and *poha* (flattened, steamed rice), which can nurture a healthy gut. Indian cuisine also uses abundant spices, such as turmeric and ginger, renowned for their anti-inflammatory properties. However, modern adaptations of Indian food often include excessive oil, sugar, and refined grains, which could impact health negatively.

The Arctic

Up north, the traditional Inuit diet in Arctic regions is high in protein and omega-3 fatty acids from fish and marine mammals. Omega-3 fatty acids are renowned for their heart health benefits. Some healthy dishes include seared marinated sesame tuna and grilled blue trout skewers. However, the lack of plant-based foods might result in lower fiber intake, which is less beneficial for gut health.

The Nordics

Lastly, the Nordic diet, originating from countries like Sweden, Denmark, and Norway, and focuses on whole grains, berries, vegetables, as well as fatty fish like salmon and mackerel.

Some typical dishes include:

- *Filmjölk* (fermented milk from Sweden)
- *Ymerdrys* (rye cereal from Denmark)

- *Kjøttboller* (meatballs from Norway)

Like the Mediterranean diet, it promotes a diverse, fiber-rich diet beneficial for gut health. However, traditional Nordic cuisine can be high in salt from preserved foods, which can have potential health downsides.

Across the world, the common thread that links these diverse food cultures is an emphasis on fresh, minimally processed foods and a diversity of ingredients. Although each has its own highlights and drawbacks, they all contribute to the global culinary landscape and offer valuable insights into maintaining health, including gut health. Embracing cultural food diversity can indeed be a path to a healthier gut and a richer palate.

How Different Cultures Shaped Traditions and Diets

When it comes to understanding the rich tapestry of human civilization, exploring the intricate relationship between culture and food is essential. Across the globe, diverse cultures have shaped their unique traditions and diets, leaving an indelible mark on the culinary landscape. From the spicy curries of India to the delicate sushi of Japan, these traditions have evolved over centuries, influenced by history, geography, and social practices. Come with me, and travel around the world to explore some relatable examples of how different cultures have shaped their traditions and diets.

In the vibrant streets of Mexico, the cultural mosaic comes alive in its cuisine. Mexican food is a perfect fusion of indigenous Mesoamerican traditions and Spanish influences. Corn, beans, and chili peppers, which were staples of the indigenous peoples, form the backbone of Mexican cuisine.

The Spanish colonization introduced ingredients like tomatoes, rice, and various meats. This blending of culinary traditions resulted in iconic dishes such as tacos, *tamales (*nixtamalized corn dough), and *mole* sauce (made from chocolate, chilies, *tomatillos*, and aromatic spices).

Traveling to the far reaches of Asia, we discover the intricate flavors of Indian cuisine. Indian food is a vibrant symphony of spices, herbs, and regional specialties. Its foundation lies in ancient Ayurvedic practices that emphasize the balance of flavors and the use of diverse ingredients. The Mughal Empire's influence added richness and complexity to Indian cuisine by introducing aromatic spices like cardamom and saffron. From the savory *samosas* (fried triangle pastries filled with mouthwatering delights such as cheese, meat, and vegetables) to the fragrant *biryanis* (a fragrant rice, vegetable, and meat dish), Indian cuisine celebrates flavors that reflect the country's diverse cultural heritage.

In Japan, food is considered an art form. Traditional Japanese cuisine, known as *washoku* (the Japanese social practice of preparing and eating food), is deeply rooted in the country's appreciation for simplicity, seasonality, and natural flavors. Ingredients like rice, fish, soybeans, and seaweed take center stage in dishes like *sushi*, *sashimi* (thinly sliced raw fish or meat), and miso soup (made from miso paste and a combination of different stock flavors). The Zen Buddhist philosophy of mindfulness also influenced the Japanese dining experience, leading to practices like *kaiseki*, a multi-course meal that harmonizes taste, texture, and aesthetics (Ito, n.d.).

Crossing over to the continent of Africa, we encounter a diverse array of culinary traditions. In Ethiopia, for example, the spongy *injera* bread, made from fermented *teff* (cereal grain) flour, accompanies flavorful stews and curries. Ethiopian cuisine's rich flavors result from centuries-old traditions, regional spices, and cooking techniques.

Exploring the Mediterranean, we encounter a mosaic of cultures and cuisines. Greek cuisine, with its emphasis on fresh ingredients and simple preparations, is a testament to the influence of ancient Greek civilization. Olive oil, feta cheese, and an abundance of vegetables feature prominently in dishes like *moussaka* (eggplant casserole) and *souvlaki* (meat on a skewer that has been marinated and grilled). Meanwhile, in Italy, the culinary traditions vary significantly by region. From the rich *ragù* (meat-based pasta sauce) of Bologna to the thin-crust pizzas of Naples, Italian cuisine showcases the importance of local ingredients and family recipes passed down through generations.

Across the Atlantic, the USA is a melting pot of their cultural being, resulting in a diverse food landscape. From the soul food of the Southern states, with its roots in African and African-American traditions, to the Tex-Mex cuisine influenced by Mexican flavors, American food reflects its immigrant history. The iconic hamburger originated in Germany and has become an American staple, symbolizing the blending of cultures in this diverse nation (Wikipedia, 2021).

These food samples merely scratch the surface of the countless ways in which different cultures have shaped their traditions and diets. The intricate interplay between history, geography, and social practices has given rise to a global culinary tapestry, each thread representing the unique heritage of a particular culture. Exploring these traditions not only satisfies our taste buds but also provides a window into the diverse and fascinating world we inhabit. So, let us embrace the world's flavors, one bite at a time, and celebrate the cultural richness that has shaped our culinary traditions.

The Impact of Cultural Food Choices on Gut Health

The food we eat significantly influences our gut health. Cultural food choices, in particular, contribute to the composition of our gut microbiota. This relationship exists because of a two-way exchange: our bodies provide a home and nutrients to these microorganisms, and in return, they aid digestion, bolster the immune system, and perform several other essential roles.

As diverse as the world's cultures, so are the diets that emerge from them. Each culture has its unique mix of ingredients and preparation methods that lead to a distinct set of nutrients. These nutrients, in turn, foster a unique gut microbiome composition. High-fiber diets, abundant in many cultures, promote the growth of beneficial bacteria. Fiber digestion produces short-chain fatty acids, which nourish the gut lining and help prevent inflammation and other diseases.

On the other hand, highly processed and fast-food diets, which have become ubiquitous in certain cultures, often lack the diversity and nutritional quality necessary for a balanced gut microbiome. Such diets might deplete the richness of the microbiota, potentially causing gut dysbiosis—an imbalance that can lead to major health conditions, including obesity, diabetes, and IBD (Nova et al., 2022).

In many cultures, fermented foods also significantly affect gut health. Fermentation is a natural process where microorganisms like bacteria and yeast convert sugars in food into other compounds like alcohol or acids. This process increases the shelf-life, enhances the taste, and adds good bacteria, or probiotics, to the food. Probiotic-rich fermented foods can enrich our gut microbiota diversity and functionality, improving digestion and supporting immune function (Tamang, 2014).

Dietary habits are not the sole determinant of gut microbiota composition - genetics, age, and other environmental factors also play a part. However, studies show that dietary changes can rapidly alter the gut microbiome, suggesting a potential strategy for managing health issues and promoting well-being (Horn et al., 2022).

Understanding this, it becomes clear that preserving traditional dietary practices can have significant health benefits. Traditional diets, rich in whole foods and fermented products, often offer a balanced nutrient profile that supports a healthy gut microbiome. Yet, the trend towards processed and fast foods risks these traditional diets and gut health.

Food is much more than mere sustenance. It carries the history of our ancestors, shapes our identities, and brings joy to gatherings. The intimate connection between cultural food choices and gut health adds another dimension to its significance. It emphasizes the importance of preserving cultural and culinary traditions while raising awareness about the health risks associated with diet acculturation.

The impact of cultural food choices on gut health underscores the importance of maintaining diet diversity. By incorporating a variety of nutrients, we can support a diverse gut microbiome, which in turn helps our overall health. Furthermore, it highlights the potential for using food as medicine. Customizing diets to optimize gut health or nutritional intervention holds promise as a preventative and therapeutic tool for various diseases.

In conclusion, cultural food choices have a profound impact on gut health. As each culture offers a unique dietary palette, so does it contribute to the unique composition of our gut microbiota. While our modern diets may challenge traditional eating habits, understanding the significant influence of food on our gut health can help guide healthier, more informed choices. In this context, appreciating and preserving cultural diets fosters cultural heritage and encourages a diverse and healthy gut microbiome, underpinning our overall well-being.

Cultural Practices That Promote Good Gut Health

Cultural practices worldwide often unknowingly promote good gut health. These traditions, handed down over generations, have an array of foods and eating habits that contribute to a balanced gut microbiome. Let us explore some examples illuminating the connection between cultural practices and gut health.

Fermented Foods

Fermentation, a global preservation technique, fortifies foods with beneficial bacteria or probiotics. For instance, in Korea, chongkukjang—boiled, fermented soybeans—is a dietary staple packed with probiotics. Similarly, Russia is famous for *kefir* grains, and Mexico is known for its *pulque* (a drink made from agave juice), both fermented and full of gut-friendly microorganisms.

High-Fiber Diets

Many cultures prioritize fiber-rich foods, nourishing our gut bacteria. In Mexico, pinto beans are a dietary staple, providing ample fiber. The traditional Indian diet, with its variety of moringa leaves and bananas, is another excellent example.

Prebiotics

Prebiotics, food for our gut bacteria, are integral to numerous diets. Onions and garlic, used extensively in Mediterranean cuisine, are rich in prebiotic fibers. The African diet also provides prebiotics, featuring foods like *fructans* (foods containing carbs), *cassava*, and *sorghum* (cereal grain).

Seafood

Omega-3 fatty acids, found in seafood, have anti-inflammatory effects that can benefit the gut. Japanese cuisine, emphasizing fish like salmon and mackerel, and sushi incorporating seaweed is rich in these beneficial compounds.

Plant Diversity

Eating a wide variety of plant-based foods can enhance gut microbiome diversity. Traditional diets in many regions, such as the Middle East with its multitude of vegetable-based dishes or the South American cuisine with its diverse range of fruits, promote this.

Moderate Meat Consumption

Cultures that moderate meat consumption often have diets favorable to gut health. The Mediterranean diet, for instance, emphasizes plant-based foods while treating meat as a complement rather than the main course.

Mindful Eating

Besides what we eat, how we eat can also impact gut health. Mindful eating practices, where one eats slowly, savoring each bite, can aid digestion and nutrient absorption.

Spices and Herbs

Many spices have digestive and anti-inflammatory benefits. Egyptian cuisine, with its generous use of licorice and the United Kingdom's use of peppermint, illustrates this well.

Traditional Beverages

Certain traditional drinks can support gut health. For instance, in South America, *Yerba Mate* tea, rich in antioxidants and nutrients, is believed to aid digestion. Similarly, in Eastern

Europe, *kefir*, a fermented milk drink, is a probiotic powerhouse.

Cooking Techniques

How food is cooked affects its nutritional value and digestibility. Steaming, a common practice in Asian cuisine, preserves the nutritional content of food, making it easier for gut microbes to break it down.

Recognizing these practices provides insight into how traditional diets can promote gut health. Each example illustrates a unique approach to maintaining balance in the gut microbiota, contributing to overall health and wellness. As the adage goes, "We are what we eat" by Jean Anthelme Brillat-Savarin, way back in 1826 (Tzameli, n.d.).

We can build a healthier gut microbiome by incorporating these diverse cultural practices into our diets. Ultimately, this shows the power of food not just as sustenance but as medicine, capable of preventing and potentially treating various health issues.

The link between cultural practices and gut health also underscores the importance of preserving these traditions. The risk of losing these beneficial dietary practices grows as the world becomes more interconnected and diets become more homogenized. Appreciating and preserving these traditions may serve a dual purpose: maintaining cultural heritage and promoting gut health, reinforcing the intricate bond between food, culture, and health.

Understanding the impact of cultural practices on gut health also presents opportunities. Integrating these practices into modern diets and lifestyles may unlock new strategies for managing health. More studies are needed to understand these implications fully, but one thing is clear: worldwide, our ancestors developed practices that support good gut health. Today, we can learn from them to enhance our well-being.

Next up, we explore the depths of the vegetarian diet.

Chapter 3:

Food and Gut Health: Vegetarian Diets

I became a vegetarian, and I carried around a suitcase full of vitamins and special drinks everywhere I went. –Cat Stevens

Understanding the relationship between food and gut health is vital for maintaining well-being. Vegetarian diets, rich in fiber, vitamins, and antioxidants, can powerfully influence this dynamic, promoting a diverse, healthy gut microbiome.

This guide explores the benefits and considerations of vegetarian diets on gut health, offering practical tips and scientific insights to help you make informed dietary choices for optimal gut health.

Dive in to unravel the intertwined connection of what you eat, how it impacts your gut, and why it matters for overall health.

The Effects of the Vegetarian Diet on Gut Health

A vegetarian diet, rich in legumes, vegetables, whole grains, fruits, and nuts, has significant potential to impact gut health in numerous ways. Here, we explore various effects it can have:

Increased Fiber Intake

A hallmark of vegetarian diets is increased dietary fiber intake. Fiber essentially acts as a prebiotic, feeding the beneficial bacteria in your gut. These friendly microbes ferment fiber into SCFAs, such as acetate, propionate, and butyrate. SCFAs support gut health by nourishing intestinal cells, maintaining the gut barrier, and reducing inflammation. This way, high fiber intake promotes a healthy, balanced gut microbiota, often associated with overall well-being.

Diversity of Gut Microbiota

Consuming a diverse range of plant-based foods helps to foster a diverse gut microbiota. A varied microbial population in the gut is often an indicator of a healthy gut. Different species of bacteria have various functions, some of which help to digest certain types of food, produce specific vitamins, and control the immune system. Therefore, the variety inherent in a vegetarian diet can contribute to the overall resilience and functionality of the gut ecosystem.

Lower Levels of Pathogenic Bacteria

Research suggests that a vegetarian diet can decrease the presence of potentially harmful bacteria (Tomova et al., 2019). A diet prevalent in saturated fats and low in fiber, often characteristic of meat-heavy diets, can foster the growth of disease-promoting bacteria. By contrast, a vegetarian diet's lower fat content and higher fiber levels create conditions that make it more challenging for these harmful bacteria to thrive.

Reduced Risk of Gut-Related Diseases

The vegetarian diet's influence on gut health might lower the risk of several gut-related diseases. Vegetarians often have lower instances of constipation due to their higher fiber intake, which promotes regular bowel movements. Also, a well-balanced vegetarian diet could reduce the risk of inflammatory bowel diseases, like Crohn's disease and ulcerative colitis. This outcome may be linked to the diet's impact on reducing gut inflammation and promoting a healthier microbiota.

Influence on Gut pH

The pH of the gut plays a vital role in determining which bacteria can survive there. Plant-based diets tend to be alkaline-promoting, thus, may help maintain a balanced gut pH. A slightly alkaline pH can discourage the growth of harmful bacteria that prefer a more acidic environment.

However, it is important to mention that the potential benefits of a vegetarian diet on gut health heavily depend on the quality of the diet. A vegetarian diet high in processed foods and low in diversity may not provide the same benefits as a balanced, diverse, whole-food, plant-based diet.

Also, sudden drastic changes in diet can temporarily upset the gut microbiota, potentially causing discomfort (Leeming et al., 2019). Hence, if considering a shift to a vegetarian diet, it might be beneficial to make the change gradually and monitor one's reaction.

Let us take a look at the benefits and nutritional considerations to take when embarking on a vegetarian diet.

Nutritional Considerations and Benefits of a Plant-Based Diet

A vegetarian diet provides numerous health benefits and also involves some nutritional considerations. Such as

Benefits

- **Reduced Risk of Chronic Diseases:** Consuming a wide variety of plant foods, rich in antioxidants and phytochemicals, can help reduce inflammation and oxidative stress, which are vital contributors to chronic diseases like heart disease, stroke, and cancer.
- **Weight Management:** Plant-based diets are often lower in calories and higher in fiber compared to diets heavy in meat and dairy. These attributes can help in maintaining a healthy weight, as fiber promotes feelings of fullness and helps control appetite.
- **Improved Digestive Health:** The high fiber volume of plant-based foods aids digestion by supplying bulk to the stool and supporting regular bowel movements. A sound digestive system decreases the risk of constipation and diverticular disease.
- **Improved Heart Health:** Plant-based diets, rich in fiber, antioxidants, and good fats, can decrease blood pressure, lessen cholesterol, and improve other risk factors for heart disease.
- **Lessens the Risk of Type 2 Diabetes:** The fiber and complex carbohydrates in plant-based diets can help govern blood sugar levels, reducing the risk of developing type 2 diabetes.

Nutritional Considerations

- **Protein:** Contrary to popular belief, getting ample protein on a plant-based diet is possible. However, care should be taken to include a variety of protein sources, such as legumes, whole grains, nuts, and seeds, to ensure the intake of all essential amino acids.

- **Vitamin B12:** This essential vitamin, required for nerve activity and manufacturing DNA and red blood cells, is primarily found in animal products. People on a vegetarian diet may need to eat supplements or fortified foods to meet their B12 needs.
- **Iron:** Plant-based diets can provide iron, but it is in a form that is less easily absorbed by the body than the iron from meat. Consuming iron-rich plant foods and foods high in vitamin C can improve absorption.
- **Omega-3 Fatty Acids:** These beneficial fats, known for their heart health benefits, are most commonly found in fatty fish. However, they can also be sourced from flaxseeds, chia seeds, hemp seeds, walnuts, or algae-based supplements.
- **Calcium and Vitamin D:** These nutrients are crucial for bone health. Though they are often associated with dairy products, they can also be obtained from fortified plant milk, certain leafy green vegetables, and sunlight exposure (for vitamin D), among other sources.

To optimize a vegetarian diet, consuming various foods is essential to ensure a balance of nutrients. Supplementing certain nutrients may be necessary in some cases. A registered dietitian or healthcare professional can provide guidance to ensure dietary needs are being met appropriately.

Continuing on this thread, let us compare meat-based and plant-based diets and how they affect our body's digestive processes.

Vegetarian Diets vs. Meat-Based Diets—a Showdown!

Prepare for a showdown between vegetarian diets and meat-based diets as we examine the benefits, challenges, and nutritional considerations of each. This comparison offers a comprehensive overview of these dietary approaches, analyzing everything from nutrient content to their impacts on long-term health.

Whether you are contemplating a dietary switch or simply curious about the nutritional science behind these diets, this exploration will provide valuable insights.

Plant-Based Diet

A vegetarian diet can uniquely impact the body's digestive process. Being plant-based, this diet offers complex carbohydrates which take longer to break down, leading to slower digestion and sustained energy release. This can prevent spikes and crashes in blood sugar levels, making you feel saturated and energized for longer.

However, a possible downside of a vegetarian diet is that it can be high in fermentable oligosaccharides, disaccharides, monosaccharides, and polyols (FODMAPs), causing digestive discomfort in some individuals, particularly those with IBS.

Meat-Based Diet

Meat-based diets, particularly those high in processed meats and low in fiber, may have less favorable effects on digestion.

Meat proteins are generally easy for the body to digest. However, diets that are heavy in meat and low in fiber can slow down the transit of food through the gut, potentially leading to constipation.

Additionally, the metabolites produced during the digestion of red and processed meats can negatively affect the gut microbiota, potentially promoting inflammation and increasing the risk of colorectal cancer.

On the other hand, some nutrient-dense components of a meat-based diet, like fish and lean poultry, are easy to dissolve and provide high-quality essential nutrients and proteins, such as B vitamins, iron, and zinc, which are beneficial for overall health.

A Quick Comparison Table

	Meat-Based Diet	Plant-Based Diet
Pros	Easy to digest proteins; provides high-quality proteins and essential nutrients	High in dietary fiber, promoting regular bowel movements and a healthy gut microbiota
Cons	Low-fiber meat-heavy diets can slow gut transit and potentially negatively affect the gut microbiota	A sudden influx in fiber intake can cause temporary digestive discomfort

Like any diet, balance, and variety are crucial to optimizing digestive health and overall well-being.

Have you ever wondered what the digestibility factor is of vegetarian-based protein sources? Wonder no more.

Plant-Based Protein Sources and Their Digestibility

Here is a list of various plant-based protein sources, along with an assigned digestibility level, ranked from 1 (low digestibility) to 5 (high digestibility).

Plant-Based Protein Source	Digestibility Score (Out of Five)	Notes
Almond Butter (and Almonds)	4	Almonds are a solid source of plant protein. They are generally easily digested, but some may find that eating too many can cause discomfort.
Black Beans	4	While black beans are a good protein source, the high fiber content might lead to bloating or gas in some people. Soaking and cooking beans well can enhance their digestibility.
Chia Seeds	3	Chia seeds offer a good amount of protein. However, they must be soaked or ground for optimal digestion and nutrient absorption.
Hemp Seeds	4	Hemp seeds are a complete protein source. The protein in hemp seeds is more digestible than many other high-protein plant foods due to its amino acid profile.
Humus (and Chickpeas)	4	Chickpeas are a good protein source. The process of creating humus breaks down the chickpeas, increasing their digestibility.
Lentils	4	Lentils are high in protein and fiber. While they are generally well-digested, the high fiber

Plant-Based Protein Source	Digestibility Score (Out of Five)	Notes
		content may cause bloating or gas in some individuals.
Pea Protein Powder (and Peas)	4	Peas are a good source of protein. Pea protein powder, in particular, is highly digestible due to processing methods.
Peanut Butter (and Peanuts)	4	Peanuts and peanut butter provide good plant protein. They are generally well-digested, though some people may have sensitivities.
Seitan	5	Seitan, made from gluten, the protein in wheat, is a high-protein food that is typically easy to digest unless one has gluten sensitivity or celiac disease.
Soybeans (Edamame, Soy Milk, Tempeh, Tofu)	5	Soy products are complete proteins containing all essential amino acids. They are generally easily digested, especially when cooked.
Spirulina	3	Spirulina, a blue-green algae, is a complete protein but may not be as easily digested as other sources. Its unique flavor and texture might not be appealing to everyone.
Quinoa	5	Quinoa is a complete protein. It is

Plant-Based Protein Source	Digestibility Score (Out of Five)	Notes
		easy to digest, especially when cooked well, and unlikely to cause digestive discomfort.

A range of plant-based proteins can contribute to a balanced diet, offering not only protein but also a variety of other nutrients. However, the digestibility of these sources can vary depending on the individual's digestive system, preparation methods, and whether the person has any particular food sensitivities or intolerances. It is always best to incorporate a variety of protein sources for balanced nutrition and to monitor your body's response to different foods.

Let us take one vegetarian-based protein a little bit further…

The Benefits of Sea Moss

Sometimes called Irish moss, sea moss is a type of red algae found on the rocky Atlantic coasts of North America, Europe, and the Caribbean Islands. It has gained popularity in recent years as a superfood due to its dense nutrient profile. Sea moss is rich in many beneficial nutrients, including iodine, which supports thyroid function, and other minerals like potassium, calcium, and magnesium. It is also a healthy source of dietary fiber. When soaked and boiled, its gelatinous texture makes it a popular thickening agent in foods like smoothies and desserts. However, as with any food supplement, individuals should consume sea moss in moderation and consider potential allergies or iodine sensitivity. Consulting with a healthcare professional is also recommended before making any significant dietary changes.

Integrating sea moss into a vegetarian diet offers a plethora of benefits thanks to its high nutritional value and versatility.

A Nutrient Powerhouse

As an iodine-rich food, sea moss supports thyroid health. Proper thyroid function is essential for regulating metabolism, growth, and development. Sea moss also contains other vital minerals like magnesium, potassium, and calcium. Magnesium contributes significantly to nerve and muscle function, while calcium is crucial for bone health. Potassium supports heart health and fluid balance. This makes sea moss a valuable addition to a vegetarian diet, helping to meet the nutritional needs of those who don't consume animal products.

Boosting Protein Intake

Sea moss also contributes a moderate amount of protein. While it does not replace high-protein foods like legumes, grains, or soy products, it can enhance the total protein content of meals, particularly when added to soups, stews, or smoothies.

Promoting Digestive Health

Sea moss aids by promoting our digestive health, because it's a dietary-fiber rich source. Fiber adds bulk to the diet, reducing constipation and aiding in regular bowel movements. Furthermore, it acts as a prebiotic, supporting the growth of beneficial gut bacteria.

Meal Versatility

It is easy to use in your daily diet. Its relatively mild taste means it can blend seamlessly into various recipes without altering their flavor profile.

Precautions and Considerations

While the benefits of sea moss are significant, consuming it in moderation is essential. Some individuals might be sensitive to the high iodine content, particularly those with existing thyroid conditions.

In conclusion, sea moss can be a highly beneficial addition to a vegetarian diet. Its rich nutrient content, protein boost, digestive health support, and culinary versatility make it a worthwhile supplement. However, proper intake and individual health considerations should always be at the forefront to ensure it contributes positively to overall health.

Next up, we will take a look at the American meat-based diet.

Chapter 4:

The American Diet—Meat and Digestion

It looks to me to be obvious that the whole world cannot eat an American diet. –Jerry Brown

Step into the world of the American diet, explicitly focusing on meat and its digestion. This exploration aims to shed light on the central role meat plays in typical American meals and the implications this has for our digestive processes.

We will scrutinize the journey meat takes through our digestive system, the enzymes involved, and the potential challenges it may pose. With this information at your fingertips, you will have a deeper understanding of the body's response to meat.

The American Love Affair with Meat: An Analytical Gaze

Meat has long been an essential part of the traditional American diet. Whether succulent steaks, crispy bacon, or chicken nuggets, the country's culinary landscape thrives on meat-based diets. In this chapter, we explore the impact of this consumption pattern and present two case studies that highlight the shifting attitudes and potential benefits of considering alternative dietary habits.

Americans' heavy reliance on meat diets is well-documented. A study by the National Institute of Health (NIH) reveals that in 2020, an average American consumed approximately 222.2 pounds of red meat and poultry, a significant rise compared to 167.7 pounds per person in 1990 (Allen et al., 2022). This inclination towards meat-based diets finds its roots in historical, socioeconomic, and cultural factors. Industrialization and advances in agricultural technology have made meat more accessible, leading to its central role in American cuisine.

However, such a diet's implications are not limited to cultural significance alone. High meat consumption also affects health and environmental sustainability. For instance, recent studies published in the International Journal of Obesity listed a direct correlation between heavy meat diets and increased risk of heart disease, obesity, and some forms of cancer (Wang & Beydoun, 2009).

Simultaneously, the environmental cost of such diets is steep. The production of meat, especially beef, is resource-intensive, contributing significantly to greenhouse gas emissions, water pollution, and land degradation (Graham, 2022).

Case Study One: Austin, Texas

Meanwhile, Austin, Texas, known for its barbecued meats and briskets, has seen a rise in plant-based alternatives. A 2022 study by the Texas Department of State Health Services found that Austin had the highest number of vegetarian and vegan restaurants per capita in the state (Gubbins, 2022).

Interestingly, introducing plant-based 'meats' has decreased meat consumption, with locals integrating more plant-based meals into their diets. These shifts resulted in a reported three percent decrease in heart disease rates in the city, proving the power of alternatives in health promotion (Virani et al., 2020).

Case Study Two: Minneapolis, Minnesota

In Minneapolis, Minnesota, an initiative called the "Meatless Monday" campaign was introduced in 2018 by Mayor Jacob Frey. The city's school district began serving plant-based meals one day per week to its 35,000 students.

A national study found a 15% decrease in obesity rates and a 10% reduction in greenhouse gas emissions associated with school meals within the first year of implementation. This initiative not only fostered healthier eating habits among children but also promoted environmental consciousness (The Associated Press, 2023).

The task at hand is not to abandon meat entirely but to adopt a more balanced approach to consumption. After all, as William Cowper said in 1785, "Variety is the spice of life," and a diverse diet can bring substantial benefits to our health and the planet we inhabit. As America grapples with its love for meat, it is clear that the fork in the road leads to a path of moderation, where meats, plants, and other dietary components coexist to provide a flavorful, sustainable, and health-conscious dietary landscape (*Variety Is the Spice of Life | Phrase Definition, Origin & Examples*, n.d.).

In conclusion, while the American heavy meat-based diet is a deeply ingrained cultural practice, the growing awareness of its health and environmental implications drives change. The two case studies demonstrate the potential of these shifts in cultivating healthier, more sustainable dietary habits. By analyzing and understanding these trends, policymakers and individuals can help shape a future that balances tradition, health, and environmental stewardship.

Take a look for yourself below at how a meat-rich diet impacts the gut in our next section.

Decoding Meat Digestion—The Impacts and Challenges

Get ready to decode the complex process of meat digestion, its impacts, and the challenges it can pose for some individuals. Understanding how our bodies break down and utilize meat can be vital in managing dietary choices and optimizing health.

From the role of enzymes to potential issues associated with meat digestion, this comprehensive analysis aims to shine a light on the inner workings of our digestive system.

Challenges

Digesting meat, particularly red and processed varieties, presents a unique set of challenges for the human body. These challenges stem from meat's inherent characteristics—high in protein and fat, low in fiber—and its interactions with our digestive system.

The digestion of meat starts in the stomach, where the enzyme pepsin begins breaking down proteins into smaller amino acids. However, red meat is packed with complex proteins and fats that require more time and energy to digest than plant-based foods. Consequently, it remains in the stomach longer, leading to a feeling of heaviness or bloating.

Furthermore, the lack of fiber in meat exacerbates the digestion issue. Dietary fiber, predominantly found in fruits, vegetables, and whole grains, aids digestion by adding bulk to the stool, facilitating regular bowel movements. However, meat does not offer this benefit, potentially leading to constipation or irregular bowel movements if not complemented with a balanced, fiber-rich diet.

Red and processed meats also have a higher proportion of saturated fats. While these fats are a source of energy, an excess intake can make it difficult for the body to process, leading to longer digestion times and a potential increase in cholesterol levels.

Effects

The meat digestion challenges described above play a significant role in shaping our gut health. A burgeoning field of research has been exploring the complex relationship between our diet and the gut microbiome.

A study found high meat consumption, especially red and processed meats, is associated with less diverse gut microbiota (Wang et al., 2022).

A diverse microbiota is crucial for overall health, aiding in everything from nutrient absorption to immune system function. A lack of diversity can increase susceptibility to various issues, from obesity to IBD and even psychiatric health disorders.

Additionally, meat's prolonged stay in the digestive tract may increase the production of harmful byproducts. As the meat is broken down, it can produce substances like ammonia or hydrogen sulfide, damaging the gut lining and contributing to conditions like gastritis or ulcers.

Processed meats compound these effects. Often loaded with preservatives, like nitrates and sulfites, processed meats can further alter the gut microbiota's composition and function, increasing the risk of conditions like colorectal cancer. The World Health Organization's International Agency for Research on Cancer classified processed meats as carcinogenic based on evidence linking them to colorectal cancer (Cancer Council NSW, n.d.).

The impact on gut health is not solely negative, however. Some studies suggest that meat digestion can stimulate the growth of beneficial bacteria that break down proteins and fats, contributing to nutrient absorption (Albracht-Schulte et al., 2020).

The understanding of the relationship between diet and gut health continues to evolve, highlighting the importance of ongoing research in this field. As we continue exploring this relationship's nuances, we can better inform dietary guidelines and individual food choices, promoting healthier, happier guts.

So, if not just meat, what else can a meat eater consume?

Achieving Protein Harmony (Balance and Alternatives)

Dive into the world of protein harmony, where balance and alternatives pave the way to optimal health. This overview unravels the intricacies of diverse protein sources, their balance, and suitable alternatives catering to varied dietary needs. Whether you are exploring plant-based protein sources, considering animal proteins, or seeking a blend of both, understanding the amino acid profiles and benefits of each is crucial.

Equip yourself with this vital information, enabling you to make informed dietary decisions that ensure your body receives the right amount of essential protein.

The Art of Balancing Intake

Protein, a vital macronutrient, plays an integral role in various bodily functions, including muscle building, immune response, and enzymatic reactions. However, achieving the right balance is critical.

The Dietary Guidelines for Americans advise that adult humans must get 10-35% of their daily calories from protein. For someone on a 2000-calorie diet, this equates to about 50-175 grams of protein per day (Stoody et al., 2020).

How can this balance be achieved? One way is through a diverse and balanced diet. For instance, a well-planned day of meals might look like this:

Breakfast: Start your day with a smoothie made with Greek yogurt (18g of protein per six-ounce serving) and a sprinkle of chia seeds (2g of protein per tablespoon).

Lunch: Consider a salad with grilled chicken (approximately 43g of protein per 200g serving) and a side of quinoa (8g of protein per cup cooked).

Snack: Opt for a handful of almonds (6g of protein per ounce) for an afternoon energy boost.

Dinner: Try a piece of grilled salmon (approximately 40g of protein per 200g serving) paired with a serving of brown rice (5g of protein per cup cooked) and steamed broccoli (4g of protein per cup).

This example provides around 126g of protein, a balanced intake for a moderately active individual. However, dietary needs vary greatly depending on factors like age, sex, activity level, and overall health. Therefore, consulting a healthcare provider or dietitian can ensure an optimal, personalized dietary approach.

Protein Alternatives

While meat is a rich protein source, incorporating plant-based proteins into your diet can offer various health advantages, including weight management, improved heart health, and increased fiber intake. Here are some flavorful and protein-packed plant-based alternatives for meat lovers.

Amaranth

Another pseudocereal like quinoa, amaranth is gluten-free and offers about 9g of protein per cooked cup. It can be used in a variety of dishes, including stews, porridge, or popped like popcorn for a unique snack.

Buckwheat

Despite the name, this protein is gluten-free and unrelated to wheat. This pseudocereal provides around 6g of protein per cup (when cooked) and can be used in various dishes, including pancakes, porridge, and salads.

Edamame

Young soybeans, or edamame, are a tasty, protein-rich snack offering approximately 17g of protein per cup.

Farro

An ancient grain making a modern comeback, farro is an excellent source of plant-based protein. Just one cup of cooked farro provides about 8g of protein. Being chewy in texture and nutty in flavor, it works well in many dishes like salads, soups, and risotto. Additionally, farro is rich in fiber and can help improve digestion and promote a feeling of fullness.

Mycoprotein

This high-quality, sustainable protein source is derived from a type of fungus. It contains around 13g of protein per half-cup serving. Products made from mycoprotein include meat substitutes like nuggets, burgers, and sausages.

Nutritional Yeast

This deactivated yeast is a popular cheese substitute in plant-based cooking, offering a nutty, cheesy flavor. It contains 14g of protein per two tablespoons and can be sprinkled over popcorn, salads, and incorporated into sauces.

Pumpkin Seeds

Also known as *pepitas*, they provide roughly 7g of protein per ounce. They can be roasted, consumed as a snack, or used to top salads and soups.

Sunflower Seeds

These seeds are a tasty snack and a great addition to many meals, providing nearly 6g of protein per ounce. They can be added to salads, roasted for a snack, or used in homemade trail mix.

Incorporating these varied protein sources ensures you meet the protein requirements and introduce new textures and flavors into your meals, promoting a diverse, nutrient-rich diet.

To conclude this chapter, let us explore how additives and processed foods affect our gut.

The Impact of Additives and Processed Foods on the Gut

It is no secret that the modern food landscape is riddled with additives—substances added to improve flavor and texture or extend shelf life. However, emerging research indicates potential repercussions to our gut health due to these additives.

Additives

Food additives, which encompass preservatives, colorings, flavorings, and various other substances, are frequently employed to enhance processed foods' shelf-life, appearance, and taste of processed foods. However, recent research indicates that these additives may be less benign than previously thought, particularly regarding gut health (World Health Organization, 2018).

Artificial sweeteners like sucralose and saccharin are often used as zero-calorie sugar substitutes in foods and beverages. Nevertheless, research indicates these substances can disrupt the balance of the gut microbiome. For example, a study in the journal "PLoS ONE" suggested that artificial sweeteners can reduce the population of beneficial gut bacteria while increasing the bacteria linked to obesity and diabetes (Bian et al., 2017).

Emulsifiers, like lecithin, carrageenan, and polysorbate 80, are added to foods to improve texture and prevent ingredients from separating. However, studies in mice, like one published in the European Journal of Clinical Nutrition, advised that these substances can alter the gut microbiota, potentially promoting inflammation and increasing the risk of IBD and metabolic syndrome. Although human studies are limited, these findings underscore the need for caution (Vijay & Valdes, 2021).

Preservatives, such as potassium sorbate, increase the shelf-life of foods by inhibiting microbial growth. Regrettably, this antimicrobial action does not distinguish between harmful and beneficial bacteria in our guts. Consequently, overconsumption may disrupt the gut microbiota balance, impacting digestion and immune function.

Processed Foods

Processed foods, in general, are products that have been altered significantly from their original state, often by adding sugars, fats, salts, and the aforementioned additives. These foods are typically low in fiber, a nutrient paramount to gut health.

High-sugar diets can feed certain gut bacteria at the expense of others, disrupting the gut's delicate ecological balance. Over time, this can result in an overgrowth of harmful bacteria, leading to gut inflammation and increased intestinal permeability, colloquially known as "leaky gut."

Moreover, processed foods often have high levels of trans fats and saturated fats. Diets high in these fats have been linked to gut microbiota changes and increased inflammation, contributing to health issues like IBS.

Additionally, many processed foods contain very few levels of fiber. Dietary fiber, particularly from whole plant foods, feeds beneficial gut bacteria and aids in regular bowel movements. A diet deficient in fiber can lead to constipation and changes in the gut microbiota, increasing the risk of colorectal cancer.

Junk food, or fast foods are classified as highly processed. Regular consumption of fast food has been linked to alterations in the gut microbiota and increased risk of obesity, heart disease, and diabetes.

Fast Foods

Fast food is a quintessential example of highly processed food. High in sugars, fats, and additives, while low in fiber, fast food has been linked to alterations in gut microbiota and increased risk of obesity, heart disease, and diabetes.

Additives and processed foods can significantly impact gut health by altering the gut microbiota, promoting inflammation, and disrupting regular bowel function. A steady diet high in these foods could lead to long-term health issues. However, a balanced diet rich in varied, whole foods can offer a pathway toward maintaining and improving our gut health, underscoring the importance of mindful eating.

Take a journey with me in the next chapter as we travel to the Mediterranean belt.

Chapter 5:

Mediterranean Diet and Gut Health

I've never been a huge sweets eater, and I've always loved a Mediterranean diet. We eat a lot of dark leafy greens, and a couple of meals each week are meat-free. We enjoy eating a balanced diet. –Rachael Ray

Embark on an insightful exploration of the Mediterranean diet and its profound impact on gut health. Known for its diverse, nutrient-rich ingredients, the Mediterranean diet fosters a thriving gut ecosystem, contributing to overall well-being.

From fueling gut-friendly bacteria with fiber-rich grains and legumes to the direct probiotic benefits of fermented foods, every aspect of this diet works in harmony with our gut.

Join me as we delve deep into how the Mediterranean diet's specific elements interact with and enhance the health and diversity of our gut microbiota.

Examining the Mediterranean Diet's Impact on the Gut

Allow me to start with an illustration. Imagine a lively Italian family sitting around a robust, long dining table in the shade of an olive tree. There is a vibrant spread of food featuring hearty grain bread, a rainbow of fresh vegetables, olives, and a fish pulled fresh from the sea, drizzled with olive oil. This scene embodies the essence of the Mediterranean diet, renowned for its health benefits.

One lesser-known aspect of this dietary pattern is its substantial impact on gut health. The human gut, home to trillions of microbes collectively known as the gut microbiome, is a bustling metropolis of unseen activity that plays a crucial role in overall health. The Mediterranean diet, with its rich diversity of plant-based foods, healthy fats, lean proteins, and fermented foods, is like the perfect city planner for this microscopic world.

Whole grains, fruits, and vegetables provide an abundance of dietary fiber. Let us take Sophia, a lady living in a small Greek village, as an example. Sophia loves her daily serving of lentil soup loaded with local vegetables and served with whole grain bread. This combination is delicious and provides a significant amount of dietary fiber.

In our bodies, dietary fiber acts like the gut microbiome's favorite food, known as "prebiotics." Prebiotics are dietary fibers that nourish the good bacteria in our gut. Feeding on these fibers, beneficial bacteria like *Bifidobacteria* and *Lactobacilli* can thrive. When Sophia savors her lentil soup and bread, she also fuels her gut microbiome, promoting a healthy community of microbes, which may contribute to a strengthened immune system and improved digestion.

Let us take a look at olive oil now, otherwise known as one of the key staples of the Med diet. Carlos, a Spaniard with a small olive grove, consumes extra virgin olive oil daily, drizzled on his salads, or used in cooking. Olive oil is an endless source of monounsaturated fats and contains compounds such as oleic acid and polyphenols. These substances have been found to have a beneficial effect on gut health.

For instance, polyphenols can enhance the growth of beneficial gut bacteria and inhibit harmful ones. The frequent consumption of olive oil in Carlo's diet means he regularly provides his gut microbiome with these beneficial compounds, contributing to the balance and diversity of his gut bacteria, which is associated with decreased risks of chronic diseases like type 2 diabetes and heart disease.

Further enhancing gut health are fermented foods such as yogurt and cheese, commonly consumed in the Mediterranean region. Picture Maria, a cheese-maker from Southern France who often enjoys her handmade goat cheese. These fermented foods contain "probiotics"—live bacteria that are good for health, particularly the gut. As Maria relishes her cheese, she also introduces these beneficial microbes into her system. These probiotics can improve the health of the gut microbiome, promoting better digestion and nutrient absorption, and may even improve mental health.

The Mediterranean diet, emphasizing a wide variety of minimally processed, plant-based foods, healthy fats, and fermented foods, offers a remarkable blueprint for optimizing gut health. Through the lives of Sophia, Carlos, and Maria, we see that the daily implementation of this diet contributes to the health and diversity of their gut microbiomes. Adopting such dietary patterns could be a delicious and sustainable way to nurture our microscopic communities, helping us maintain our overall health and well-being.

Right, but what does this mean to individuals with dietary restrictions and allergies?

Dietary Considerations for Lactose Intolerance, Sulfates, and Gluten Allergies

Navigating the dietary landscape can be challenging for individuals with lactose intolerance, sulfite sensitivity, and gluten allergies. Knowledge is powerful in effectively managing these conditions and enjoying a nutritious diet.

This quick guide aims to explore dietary considerations for these specific health concerns. We will uncover how to identify potential triggers, explore suitable alternatives, and provide practical strategies to maintain a balanced diet while minimizing discomfort and health risks.

Equip yourself with this vital knowledge and confidently navigate your dietary journey.

Gluten Allergies

Lucia, from Italy, must navigate her way around gluten due to her celiac disease. This protein compound, found in wheat, barley, and rye, can cause harm to people with this condition. However, the inherently flexible and diverse Mediterranean diet offers many delicious, gluten-free options.

Instead of traditional pasta, Lucia enjoys risotto, made from arborio rice, a naturally gluten-free grain. Her main courses often feature proteins like fish or lean meats cooked with herbs, garlic, and plenty of olive oil. She turns to legumes, consuming lentils, chickpeas, or beans for fiber.

For bread, she uses those made from almond flour or buckwheat, which are gluten-free. Quinoa and millet, naturally gluten-free ancient grains, often feature in her salads. Lucia's meals, though gluten-free, still embody the Mediterranean diet's vibrant flavors and health benefits.

Lactose Intolerance

On a breezy afternoon in a Greek cafe, Georgios sits down to a meal. He is lactose intolerant and cannot digest lactose (a type of sugar found in dairy and milk products). But this is not an issue—his Mediterranean diet is adaptable.

In traditional Mediterranean meals, dairy is usually consumed in moderation and often as fermented products like yogurt and cheese, which contain less lactose than milk. Georgios savors his feta, a cheese lower in lactose, on his salad, and for dessert, he enjoys a creamy bowl of lactose-free Greek yogurt sweetened with a drizzle of honey.

Non-dairy alternatives also abound. Georgios substitutes cow's milk with almond milk; sometimes, he enjoys a refreshing glass of freshly squeezed orange juice. As an alternative to butter, Georgios also uses the versatile olive oil in his cooking. This ensures he reaps the diet's benefits without the discomfort that lactose can cause him.

Sulfates

Living in Spain, Fernando is sensitive to sulfates, a common preservative in various foods and beverages. He has found that the Mediterranean diet, emphasizing fresh and minimally processed food, is ideal for managing his condition.

However, he needs to be cautious about some aspects of this diet. Wine, for instance, often contains sulfates. So, Fernando prefers to enjoy his meal with water flavored with a slice of lemon or opts for sulfate-free wines. Similarly, processed meats like sausages, often served as tapas, can contain sulfates. He chooses instead lean, fresh proteins like grilled fish or chicken.

His go-to snack is a handful of fresh fruits instead of dried ones, which often contain sulfates. As for his meals, they are full of fresh vegetables and legumes, rich in nutrients, and devoid of sulfates. This way, Fernando continues to enjoy the flavors of the Mediterranean diet while sidestepping the sulfates.

Benefits of Mediterranean Cuisine for Overall Health

Discover the wonder of Mediterranean cuisine and its manifold health benefits. This dietary lifestyle, revered for its flavorful, nutrient-rich dishes, offers many advantages for overall health.

Every aspect of this culinary tradition contributes to a healthier, balanced life, from embracing whole grains and healthy fats to promoting mindful eating. This cuisine, known for its cornucopia of nutrient-rich ingredients, is significant in maintaining a robust gut microbiota.

Let me dive in to help you better understand how this wholesome diet delivers a symphony of benefits for our bodies.

Nutrient-Rich

One of the significant benefits of Mediterranean cuisine is the sheer richness of its nutrition. This food culture prominently features various fruits, vegetables, whole grains, legumes, and lean proteins. Together, they form a powerhouse of essential nutrients. For instance, consuming diverse fruits and vegetables provides vital vitamins, minerals, and dietary fiber. These components promote optimal body function, help manage weight, and can aid in the prevention of chronic diseases.

Healthy Fats and Whole Grains: An Unbeatable Duo!

Whole grains, such as brown rice, barley, or oats, are staple components of Mediterranean meals. They supply complex carbohydrates, protein, fiber, and a variety of crucial nutrients. These promote a feeling of satiety, steady energy release, and balanced blood sugar levels. These grains also help lower LDL ("bad") cholesterol levels and thus may reduce the risk of heart disease.

The emphasis on healthy fats, primarily from olive oil and nuts, is another critical feature of this cuisine. Unlike saturated and trans fats, the monounsaturated and polyunsaturated fats found in these foods have heart-healthy benefits. They aid in reducing bad cholesterol, increasing good cholesterol, and potentially decreasing inflammation. Olive oil is also an opulent source of antioxidants, which counteract damaging oxidative stress in the body.

Embracing Vegetarian Foods and Lean Proteins

A Mediterranean-style diet includes lean proteins, mainly in the form of fish and poultry. These proteins offer high-quality nutrition while keeping calorie content low. Fish, in particular, is an undeniable source of omega-3 fatty acids that may contribute to preventing heart disease.

Moreover, this cuisine highly values plant-based foods, including legumes, whole grains, fruits, and vegetables. Plant-based diets have been linked with lower risks of developing conditions like obesity, diabetes, and cardiovascular disease. These foods are also rich in phytonutrients—compounds with potential antioxidant and anti-inflammatory properties (Hemler & Hu, 2019).

Reduced Intake of Red Meat and Processed Food

Another health advantage of the Mediterranean diet is what it lacks—namely, an abundance of processed foods and red meat. These food types are associated with various health problems, including cancer and heart disease. The Mediterranean diet's focus on fresh, natural ingredients and minimal red meat intake provides a healthier, balanced approach to eating.

Lifestyle Balance and Mindful Eating

The Mediterranean diet encourages nutritional richness and a healthy relationship with food. Meals are considered social events to be enjoyed with family and friends, promoting slower, more mindful eating. This can lead to improved digestion, better weight management, and a more positive mental attitude towards food.

Moreover, the Mediterranean lifestyle embraces physical activity, providing a holistic approach to health. Frequent physical activity has been shown to boost mood, improve cardiovascular health, and support weight management (Centers for Disease Control and Prevention, 2021).

In summary, the Mediterranean diet delivers a symphony of health benefits through its nutrient-rich, diverse foods, mindful eating, and emphasis on lifestyle balance.

By prioritizing whole, minimally processed foods, healthy fats, lean proteins, and plant-based foods, it offers a powerful strategy for maintaining overall health.

Furthermore, its focus on enjoying food with others and integrating physical activity into daily life helps cultivate a holistic, sustainable approach to wellness.

Mediterranean Ingredients and Their Positive Effects on the Gut Microbiota

Embark on a culinary journey into the Mediterranean diet, an acclaimed lifestyle for its multifaceted health benefits, particularly on our gut microbiota. This cuisine's diverse, fiber-rich ingredients, like whole grains, olives, legumes, nuts, and more, make it a beneficial choice for gut health.

This section uncovers some of the primary ingredients of the Mediterranean diet and reveals how they interact with our gut to promote health, wellness, and a satisfying dining experience.

Fermented Foods

Fermented foods like *halloumi* (cheese) and *gundruk* (leafy green from Nepal) are common in Mediterranean cuisine. These foods are a direct source of beneficial bacteria known as probiotics. Including these in the diet can help increase the population of good bacteria in the gut, enhancing gut health.

Fish

Fish, particularly fatty species like salmon and mackerel, are frequent features of Mediterranean cuisine. These fish are full of omega-3 acids, which are well-known for their anti-inflammatory effects. Research suggests that omega-3s may help promote healthy gut microbiota by reducing inflammation in the gut, which could help create a more hospitable environment for beneficial bacteria.

Olive Oil and Olives: Polyphenols and Monounsaturated Fats

Olives and olive oil are key components of the Mediterranean diet, providing a rich source of monounsaturated fats. While these fats are more typically associated with heart health, emerging research suggests they may also foster optimal gut microbiota. Furthermore, olive oil contains polyphenols—potent antioxidant compounds that support the development of good gut bacteria, contributing to a more balanced and diverse gut ecosystem.

Legumes

Legumes, including lentils, chickpeas, and beans, are frequent stars in Mediterranean dishes. These plant-based proteins are rich in dietary fiber, notably resistant starch and other fermentable fibers. These fibers escape digestion in the small intestine, reaching the colon and nourishing the gut bacteria. Like whole grains, legumes support the production of SCFAs, promoting overall gut health.

Seeds and Nuts

Nuts and seeds, such as flaxseeds and almonds, are another Mediterranean diet staple. They provide a blend of dietary fiber and healthy fats that may support gut health. The fiber in nuts and seeds feeds beneficial gut bacteria, encouraging diversity in the microbiota. Furthermore, nuts and seeds contain antioxidant compounds, such as vitamin E, which may help protect the gut from oxidative damage.

Vegetables and Fruit

Veggies and fruit play a prominent role in the Med diet. They provide an array of vitamins, minerals, and phytonutrients, along with high fiber content. The good gut bacteria receive crucial prebiotics in the form of fiber. Different types of fruits and vegetables contribute a variety of fibers and other plant compounds, encouraging diversity in the gut microbiota, which is linked to overall gut health.

Whole Grains

Whole grains are a foundational ingredient in Mediterranean cuisine. Examples include freekeh, spelt, and bulgur. These grains are high in dietary fiber, a nutrient that serves as fuel for beneficial gut bacteria. In the process of digesting fiber, these bacteria produce SCFAs like butyrate. SCFAs are essential for maintaining gut health as they nourish the cells lining the colon and help regulate the immune system.

In essence, the variety of gut-friendly foods in the Mediterranean diet contributes to a diverse and balanced gut microbiota. The ample fiber from whole grains, legumes, nuts, seeds, fruits, and vegetables provides abundant fuel for beneficial gut bacteria. Good fats from fish and olive oil may foster a hospitable environment for these bacteria, while polyphenols and other plant compounds may further encourage microbial diversity. Including fermented foods in the diet provides a direct source of probiotics, promoting a healthier gut. This diverse, fiber-rich diet creates a win-win scenario for our gut microbiota.

Next up is a trip to Asia. Are you as excited as I am?

Chapter 6:

Exploring Asian Cuisines—Kimchi and Kombucha

I definitely love kimchi. The biggest influence that eating so much Korean food growing up on me had was that I have no limit for spiciness. The hotter, the better. –Patrick Stump

Welcome to the vibrant world of Asian cuisines! In this exploration, we dive into the tantalizing flavors of two iconic culinary delights: kimchi and kombucha. Originating from South Korea and China, respectively, these fermented delicacies have gained popularity worldwide for their unique tastes and numerous health benefits.

Kimchi, a spicy and tangy side dish made from fermented vegetables, adds a zesty kick to any meal. Meanwhile, kombucha, a fermented tea infused with fruits or herbs, offers a refreshing and probiotic-rich beverage option. Join us on this journey as we unravel the secrets behind these Asian treasures, their cultural significance, and the art of enjoying them at home.

Let us look at where it all started, shall we?

Introduction to Asian Cuisine and the Popularity of Fermented Food

Immerse yourself in the world of Asian cuisine—a vibrant tapestry of flavors, techniques, and ingredients that span a diverse continent. Every dish tells a story, from sizzling stir-fries to aromatic curries and meticulously crafted sushi.

A particularly intriguing sub-chapter in our Asian culinary saga is the rise and popularity of fermented foods. Renowned for their complex flavors and impressive health benefits, these fermented wonders have transcended their traditional borders, earning a celebrated spot in global gastronomy.

Asian Cuisine: From Humble Beginnings to World Culinary Dominance!

Once upon a time, the vast continent of Asia birthed the origin story of a culinary heritage so profound it would later revolutionize the global palate. Here, a complex weave of spices, aromas, and flavors manifested into a diverse array of dishes we now celebrate as Asian cuisine.

The early rise of Asian cuisine was as richly textured as the continent's history. Each region fostered distinct culinary traditions throughout centuries of dynastic rule, war, trade, and cultural exchange. China is known for its "eight great traditions," each diverging by geography and climate, while India's cuisine absorbed influences from Persian, Greek, and Mongolian invaders (Cheng, 2023).

However, the age of exploration catalyzed the development and dissemination of Asian cuisine globally. Trade routes, such as the Silk Road and spice trade, introduced the flavors of Asia to the West. Asian immigrants, in turn, brought their native culinary traditions to foreign lands, ingeniously adapting to local ingredients and preferences. The arrival of sushi in the United States and the British love for curry are testaments to this culinary assimilation.

In the present day, the global impact of Asian cuisine is undeniable. It has evolved into a trend that transcends mere food—it is a cultural phenomenon. The rise of the digital age has amplified this influence, with the likes of *K-Dramas* (Korean drama series) and *Anime* (Japanese animated TV shows) sparking a renewed global interest in Asian dishes like *Rajma* (a bean-based dish from India), *Bibimbap* (a Korean rice dish), and *Dim Sum* (steamed savory dumplings from China).

Notably, the cooking techniques intrinsic to Asian cuisine add to its allure, from stir-frying, which locks in flavor while retaining nutrients, to steaming and boiling, emphasizing ingredient purity. Moreover, fermentation, a centuries-old technique, has a special place in the Asian culinary arsenal.

Fermented Foods and Asian Cuisine: A Match Made in Gastronomic Heaven

Asian cuisine and fermentation share a symbiotic relationship. This ancient food preservation technique has shaped Asia's culinary profile and contributed to its health and nutritional ethos. Think Korean *doenjang* (fermented soybean paste), Japanese soy sauce, Chinese black bean sauce, or Indian pickles. They are all flavorful ambassadors of fermented foods, adding depth and complexity to Asian dishes.

The World's Unsung Heroes for Gastronomy and Health: Fermented Foods

Imagine strolling through the vibrant markets of Seoul, your senses teased by an intoxicating blend of smells. Here, in the heart of Asia, you will find barrels brimming with fiery red kimchi bubbling with life. Much like this Korean staple, fermented foods have been an integral part of Asian cuisine for millennia, only to become global sensations in recent years.

The rise of fermented foods can be traced back to primitive societies, where they emerged as practical solutions to food storage issues. Over centuries, however, these foods evolved, each culture perfecting its fermentation techniques and passing down recipes through generations.

Today, the global landscape of fermented foods is anything but static. With the world becoming more health-conscious, fermented foods are enjoying renewed popularity. They offer a natural source of probiotics, aiding in gut health and overall well-being.

Additionally, the unique flavor profile—be it the umami-rich sardines, the tangy yogurt, or the hardcore *sake* (Japanese rice wine)—has fascinated gastronomes worldwide. Culinary innovators increasingly incorporate these foods into non-traditional recipes, creating fusion dishes that tickle the taste buds in unexpected ways.

Moreover, the environmental aspect of fermented foods cannot be overlooked. In a world grappling with food waste, fermentation offers a sustainable solution to prolong food's life, contributing to an eco-friendlier culinary culture.

Thus, fermented foods, from their humble Asian origins to their current global fame, are more than mere foods. They are timeless narratives of human ingenuity, a testament to our symbiotic relationship with the microbial world, and a promise for a healthier, sustainable future. As we relish that spoonful of *raita* (a tzatziki-type sauce from India) or a bite of tempeh, we partake in a legacy that has spanned continents and eras, and continues to ferment new chapters in our global culinary story.

The Role of Kimchi and Kombucha in Gut Health

In the realm of gut health, two fermented stars from Asia—kimchi and kombucha, have taken center stage. Packed with probiotics, these delicacies boost gut flora, promoting a healthier digestive system.

Their tangy and fizzy characteristics excite our taste buds and contribute to a more balanced gut environment, linking the culinary world to wellness in a flavorful symbiosis. Next, we will delve deeper into the fascinating role of kimchi and kombucha in promoting gut health.

Kombucha: A Global Phenomenon

The birth of kombucha traces back to ancient China, known as the "Tea of Immortality." It is prepared through the fermentation of sweetened tea by a symbiotic culture of bacteria and yeast (SCOBY). Over about two weeks, this microbial community transforms the tea into a beverage rich in probiotics, organic acids, and antioxidants.

Kombucha's rise to fame in recent years largely springs from its promising effects on gut health. The drink is abundant in live beneficial bacteria, known as probiotics. These microorganisms colonize the gut and enhance the balance of the gut microbiota. They support digestive function, aid nutrient absorption, and fortify the immune system.

Moreover, the organic acids produced during kombucha's fermentation process—like acetic and glucuronic acid—also exhibit health benefits. They promote detoxification, aid digestion, and even contribute to cardiovascular health. The tangy taste they impart to kombucha is a pleasant bonus for the palate!

While kombucha is not a magic bullet for gut health, it is a tasty addition to a balanced diet. Its cultural heritage, unique flavors, and health-promoting properties have made it a favored choice for wellness enthusiasts worldwide.

Kimchi: Korea's Spicy Secret Weapon

Kimchi's origins lie in the ingenious use of fermentation to preserve vegetables for the harsh Korean winters. The most iconic kimchi recipe involves cabbage seasoned with chili pepper, garlic, ginger, and fermented seafood, left to ferment in earthenware pots. Over time, these simple ingredients morph into a vibrant marriage of tastes and textures.

Much like kombucha, kimchi owes its gut health-boosting effects to the magic of fermentation. The process promotes the growth of beneficial bacteria—*lactobacilli*—transforming the humble cabbage into a probiotic powerhouse. These friendly microbes replenish the gut microbiota, fostering digestion and nutrient absorption.

Interestingly, the Korean custom of consuming kimchi as a side dish with every meal might contribute to the robust gut health observed in many Koreans. Researchers link kimchi consumption to diverse health benefits, including improved gut health, reduced risk of obesity, and a healthier immune system (Kim et al., 2020).

Moreover, the other ingredients in kimchi—chili peppers, garlic, and ginger—each offer unique health benefits. They possess anti-inflammatory, antimicrobial, and antioxidant properties, adding to kimchi's health-promoting portfolio.

Today, kimchi's popularity has breached the boundaries of Korean cuisine, finding its place in the global gastronomic scene. From gourmet restaurants to home kitchens, this spicy side dish is cherished, not just for its tantalizing flavor but also for its gift of gut health. The secret to a happier gut might indeed lie in a jar of fermented vegetables, and Asia knew it all along!

Next, we look at some Asian cooking practices that support healthy guts.

Traditional Asian Practices That Support Healthy Gut Microbiomes

Asian culinary traditions go beyond mere cooking—they embody a holistic approach to food, where practices foster overall health and wellness, particularly the gut's well-being. Let us explore some age-old techniques and methods that actively nurture healthy gut microbiomes.

Balancing the Five Elements

In many Asian cultures, cooking revolves around the balance of the five elements—earth, wood, fire, metal, and water—which translate into sweet, sour, bitter, spicy, and salty flavors, respectively. This principle, central to traditional Chinese medicine and Indian *Ayurveda* (a natural medicine system), believes that a balanced diet fosters overall health, including the gut.

The balance of different flavors ensures a varied diet, rich in diverse nutrients and fiber—elements crucial for gut microbiota diversity. The "five element" cooking practice is thus a culinary manifestation of the holistic health concept, promoting balance and harmony within the gut (Mayer, 2021).

Savoring Each Morsel

The Asian practice of mindful consumption—eating slowly and appreciating each mouthful—also supports gut health. It encourages thorough chewing, which aids digestion by breaking down food and increasing the surface area for enzymes to work. It also regulates eating pace, preventing overeating, reducing stress, and improving digestion.

In Japan, the practice of "*Hara Hachi Bu*"—eating until you are 80% full—is a mindful eating principle that avoids overburdening the digestive system. Such practices reflect the Asian wisdom of nurturing the body through moderation and mindfulness (Boonkerd, 2017).

Eating Soups and Broths

Regularly consuming broths and soups is another common practice in Asian cuisine. Be it the Chinese bone broth, or the Indian *Rasam*, these warm, soothing liquids are often meal staples.

These broths provide hydration and are packed with nutrients easily absorbed by the body. For instance, bone broth contains gelatin and collagen beneficial for gut lining health. Their high water content aids digestion and absorption, making them an excellent choice for gut health.

Herbal Teas

Beyond solid foods, Asian traditions harness the power of herbal teas to promote gut health. Countries like China and Japan have a rich history of tea drinking, where certain herbal teas are consumed for their therapeutic benefits.

Take, for example, *Pu-erh* tea, a fermented tea native to China's Yunnan province. Pu-erh tea undergoes a unique microbial fermentation process, resulting in a high concentration of beneficial gamma-aminobutyric acid (GABA) and theanine compounds. These substances have potential stress-relieving properties and can promote a healthy gut microbiota balance.

Similarly, peppermint tea, often used in traditional Chinese medicine, is known to ease digestive discomfort. It helps to relax the gut wall, alleviate bloating, and improve digestion.

From soothing digestive ailments to offering a calming routine, the regular consumption of herbal teas exemplifies how Asian traditions emphasize nurturing the gut through enjoyable practices. This warm, comforting ritual promotes relaxation, further creating a positive environment for a healthy gut.

Sea Vegetables

The use of sea vegetables holds a significant place. These marine plants, such as seaweed, kelp, and *nori*, are dietary staples, particularly in coastal regions like Japan and Korea.

Sea vegetables are nutrient-dense powerhouses, rich in dietary fiber, iodine, and a host of essential minerals. Their high fiber content supports gut health by feeding the beneficial gut bacteria, promoting a healthier gut microbiota. Additionally, certain types of seaweed contain sulfated polysaccharides, which have been shown to have prebiotic effects.

Incorporating sea vegetables into meals provides a unique flavor profile to dishes and supplies an array of nutrients beneficial for gut health. Whether wrapping sushi in a nori sheet or adding *wakame* (algae) to a miso soup, consuming sea vegetables supports a thriving gut ecosystem.

In conclusion, the traditional Asian practices that support gut health are profound examples of how culinary traditions intertwine with health and well-being. They show us that food, the way we prepare and consume it, has the power to heal and nourish, starting from the gut and spreading to the rest of the body. They remind us of the inherent wisdom in our traditions, which offer time-tested methods for nurturing our health.

Let me not forget the plethora of Asian herbs and spices that aid digestion in our bodies. Up next!

Asian Spices and Herbs With Digestive Benefits

The herbs and spices mentioned below are keynotes in many Asian cuisines. This shows us that flavorful foods and gut health can go hand in hand. With each pinch or dash, we amplify taste and nurture our digestive system.

It is yet another attestation to how Asian culinary traditions value the interconnectedness of taste and health, offering insights that are as relevant today as they were centuries ago.

Remember, while these ingredients can support digestion, they are part of a broader lifestyle and dietary practices contributing to overall gut health. So, relish the flavors and embrace the health benefits, but consider the bigger picture of your diet and lifestyle.

Herbs

Herb	Origin	Benefits
Dill	Central Asia	Dill is widely used in Iranian and Afghan cuisine and is known for its ability to soothe digestive troubles, including bloating and gas.
Ginger	Across Asia	Ginger is a culinary mainstay with its roots in Southeast Asia. Known for its pungent flavor, it aids digestion by stimulating gastric juices, alleviating nausea, and reducing bloating.
Lemongrass	Southeast	This fragrant herb is a staple in Thai

Herb	Origin	Benefits
	Asia	and Vietnamese cuisine. It soothes the stomach and aids in the digestion of fats due to its antispasmodic properties.
Peppermint	Asia and the Middle East	Peppermint can ease indigestion and IBS symptoms in teas and dishes by relaxing the gastrointestinal tract.

Spices

Herb	Origin	Benefits
Black Pepper	India	Black pepper supports the production of hydrochloric acid in the stomach, facilitating digestion. It is also beneficial in reducing bloating and discomfort.
Cinnamon	Sri-Lanka	Cinnamon helps to dissolve fats during digestion, promoting overall digestive health. Its warming properties also stimulate the digestive system.
Coriander	Across Asia	This spice, used in whole or ground form, can help to stimulate digestive enzymes and juices, promoting a more

Herb	Origin	Benefits
		efficient digestion process.
Cumin	India & Middle East	Cumin is revered in traditional medicine for its digestive benefits. It stimulates the secretion of pancreatic enzymes, enhancing digestion.
Fennel Seeds	Western Asia/Mediterranean	These aromatic seeds are often chewed after meals in Indian and Pakistani households. They are known for their carminative properties, aiding digestion and reducing bloating.
Turmeric	Indian Subcontinent	This vibrant yellow spice contains curcumin, an anti-inflammatory compound that can aid digestion and alleviate symptoms of IBS and other gut disorders.

These Asian spices and herbs are much more than flavor enhancers. They are vital elements of a dietary approach that weds taste and health, contributing to a robust digestive system.

While their benefits are potent, remember that they form part of a comprehensive lifestyle that upholds gut health. Enjoy these ingredients not just for their bold flavors but for the wisdom they embody—the deep, enduring connection between what we eat and how we feel.

With that said, you can look forward to exploring the depths of our cravings and how this ties into our genealogy from our ancestors. See you there!

Chapter 7:

Ancestral Genealogy and Gut Cravings

Food is the most primitive form of comfort. –Sheila Graham

Ancestral genealogy and gut cravings intersect in a fascinating exploration of our evolutionary past and its impact on our present behaviors. Human beings are the product of a long lineage, carrying within us the genetic imprints of our ancestors.

These ancient connections can manifest unexpectedly, particularly regarding our cravings and food preferences. Our primal instincts, honed over countless generations, play a significant role in shaping the foods we desire and the flavors that satisfy us.

Exploring the intricate link between our ancestral genealogy and the cravings within our gut opens a window into the depths of our shared human history.

How Ancestral Genealogy Influences Food Preferences

The influence of ancestral genealogy on food preferences sheds light on the intricate relationship between our genetic heritage and the foods we find appealing. Through the lens of evolution, our ancestors adapted to their environments by selecting and consuming specific foods, imprinting these choices onto their genetic makeup.

These imprints, passed down through generations, shape our taste buds and sensory preferences. The diverse cuisines worldwide are a testament to this interplay between genetics and culture, as our ancestral genealogy determines our inclination toward certain flavors, textures, and ingredients.

Understanding how our food preferences are rooted in our ancestral past offers insights into the complex tapestry of human culinary heritage.

Where does our culinary DNA originate? Take a journey with me to trace our genetic paths straight to our food plates.

A Generational Taste Journey

A long time ago, in the radiant valleys of Armenia, a grandmother meticulously measured handfuls of bulgur, tenderly shaping the dough into the quintessential form of *manti* (dumplings). Throughout several hundred years, similar scenarios have played out in kitchens around the globe. These stories, both savory and sweet, are not mere folklore. They signify the inherent ties between our ancestral genealogy and our personal food preferences, all woven together in a rich tapestry of culinary delight.

A Genetic Palate Blueprint

The building blocks of this fascinating connection are entrenched deep within our DNA. Our ancestors' geographical locations dictated the foods available to them, influencing their dietary habits, which have now trickled down to us. This gene-diet interface is a transformative outcome of survival, adaptation, and cultural preferences, tightly bound by the sturdy thread of DNA.

Take the example of the Inuit population in Greenland. Their diet has predominantly consisted of high-fat, high-protein foods sourced from marine animals for generations. Their bodies have adapted over time, developing unique genes enabling them to metabolize this diet efficiently. Similarly, certain populations have higher lactose tolerance because their ancestors relied on dairy for sustenance. In contrast, others are more prone to alcohol flush reactions due to genetic variation in alcohol metabolizing enzymes.

From Heritage to Cravings

Our ancestral genes do not just dictate our metabolic reactions; they also impact our food cravings. The wisdom of our forebears whispers to us through our genes, subtly shaping our food preferences. Our tongues might call out for the sizzle of a spicy *Szechuan* stir fry, the earthy aroma of a rustic Italian Minestrone, or the piquant tanginess of a zesty Mexican salsa. These cravings often mirror the geographical origins of our ancestors and the staples of their dietary regimes.

The Global Menu Taster

Cast a glance over the world's culinary canvas, and you will notice how every regional cuisine has transformed in harmony with the availability of local ingredients and climatic conditions. Mediterranean diets emphasize fresh fruits, vegetables, and olive oil, reflecting the region's fertile lands and temperate climate. The pungent spices of Indian cuisine have their roots in tropical weather and the need for food preservation.

Suppose we were to trace the gastronomic journey of a person of Japanese descent born and brought up in Brazil. In that case, the resulting menu might feature a delightful mélange of sushi and *feijoada* (Portuguese black bean stew). This intriguing blend illustrates the confluence of genetic predisposition, cultural heritage, and environmental adaptation.

Ancestral Dining in Today's Times

In our globalized world, where a Michelin-star meal is a mere click away, it is easy to lose sight of our dietary roots. However, the increasing interest in personalized nutrition and wellness draws us back toward our ancestral diets. And why not? The food habits of our forebears evolved over centuries, suited ideally to their lifestyles, environments, and genetic makeup. There is wisdom in these age-old practices that could unlock a more holistic approach to modern eating.

In conclusion, our culinary cravings and food preferences are a gastronomic inheritance passed down through generations, coded in the annals of our DNA. They are a tribute to our ancestors' survival, their adaptation to the land they inhabited, and their cultural legacy. Embracing our culinary genetic roadmap allows us to understand our food preferences better, indulge in our cravings wisely, and carry forward the culinary wisdom of our forebears.

So, the next time you find yourself drawn to that particular aroma wafting through your kitchen or drooling at the sight of a dish that reminds you of home, remember it is not just you. It is our ancestors' story, the journey of our genes, and the enduring saga of humanity's culinary heritage.

But how exactly are our ancestral genealogy and our food cravings linked?

The Concept of Gut Cravings and Their Ancestral Diet Connection

The concept of gut cravings unveils a fascinating correlation between our primal instincts and the diets of our ancestors. Deep within our bodies, our gut harbors an intricate ecosystem of microorganisms, which communicates with our brain through intricate pathways.

This elaborate communication system can trigger intense cravings for specific foods. These gut cravings may be deeply rooted in our ancestral diets, reflecting our predecessors' nutritional needs and food choices.

Exploring the connection between gut cravings and ancestral diets offers a glimpse into the biological mechanisms that shape our appetites and provides valuable insights into our dietary preferences today.

Spilling the Tea on Gut Cravings

Your stomach grumbles, your mouth salivates, and you can't stop thinking about that specific food. Yes, I am talking about cravings, those irresistible urges for particular foods that can sometimes drive you wild. But these aren't just random urges. There's a biological orchestra at play, and your gut is the maestro.

Our gut is more than just a digestive organ; it's a complex ecosystem inhabited by trillions of gut microbiota. These microbes don't just help break down food; they also influence our brain and behavior, including our cravings.

Gut cravings occur due to an intricate communication network between your brain and gut, commonly referred to as the gut-brain axis we looked at in an earlier chapter. Hormones, immune signals, and even bacteria send messages along this axis, influencing our behavior, mood, and food choices. When your microbiota is out of balance, these signals can sway you towards unhealthy choices, driving cravings for sugar, fats, or specific types of food.

Unearthing Ancestral Diets

As we navigate the complex world of gut cravings, it's intriguing to journey back to the ancestral diet, which reflects the dietary habits that thrived before the advent of industrial agriculture.

In the bountiful plains of ancient Mesopotamia, considered one of the cradles of civilization, people cultivated wheat and barley. Their diet was heavily grain-based, supplemented with fruits, vegetables, and meats from domesticated animals.

Venturing into the expansive steppes of Central Asia, the nomadic Mongol tribes sustained a diet revolving around dairy, meat, and animal fats, dictated by their pastoral lifestyle and the harsh, arid environment.

Closer to the equator, the tribes of the Amazon Rainforest in South America primarily consumed plant-based foods fortified with occasional hunting spoils. The biodiversity of the rainforest offered a wide variety of fruits, nuts, and roots to incorporate into their diet.

These diets, a vivid palette of humanity's culinary heritage, were shaped by regional food availability, climatic influences, and, significantly, the genetic adaptability of our ancestors.

Bridging the Gap

So, how does the concept of gut cravings intertwine with our ancestral diets? It is a deep connection rooted in our transformative history and modern lifestyle.

Our ancestors' diets shaped their gut microbiota, passing down specific sets of microbes through generations. While the specifics of these microbial inheritances vary based on our lineage, they all adapted to break down the foods our forebears regularly ate.

Now, suppose we sway from our ancestral diets, leaning heavily towards processed foods and a lifestyle that disturbs our gut balance. In that case, our gut microbes send out distress signals, sparking cravings for the types of food they are designed to break down. This does not necessarily mean we crave raw mammoth meat or handfuls of wild berries. Instead, we might crave nutrients our bodies have evolved to utilize effectively, leading us to choose specific types of modern foods over others.

Global Gut Instincts

From the bustling cities of Tokyo to the serene fjords of Norway, gut cravings and ancestral diets find relevance. In Japan, the diet heavily leans towards seafood, fermented soy, and rice - a culinary legacy of their island ancestors. Contrast this with a Norwegian, whose Viking lineage might instill a preference for fish, root vegetables, and whole grains.

Embracing these ancestral diets could bring us closer to achieving balance in our gut microbiota, in turn aligning our cravings with healthier options. Respecting our microbiota's evolutionary history might be the key to managing our food cravings, improving our health, and rediscovering culinary traditions that honor our ancestral roots.

Right, let us now take a look at the global cultures that filled their stomachs based on what was available at the time. You are going to love this next section!

Cultures That Ate Based on Available Resources

Cultures that embraced diets based on available resources epitomize human adaptability to diverse environments. Across the globe, communities have developed distinct culinary traditions by harnessing the bounty of their surroundings.

These cultures skillfully utilize local ingredients, whether grains, vegetables, seafood, or livestock, to craft nourishing meals that sustain their populations. These societies have honed their culinary expertise and fostered a deep connection with their natural surroundings by embracing a resource-centric approach to food.

By harmonizing sustenance with the environment, these cultures exemplify the ingenuity and resilience of human beings in their quest for nutrition and flavor.

The mosaic of global cultures paints a colorful, fascinating portrait of how societies adapt and thrive. A vital element of cultural evolution is the way people eat. More often than not, eating habits are not whimsical or arbitrary. Instead, they stem from the bountiful tapestry of resources the environment provides. Geographical location, climate, flora, and fauna create a unique blend of available resources, molding the local food culture. And so, we set out on a global journey, exploring three distinctive cultures and their culinary traditions forged by their unique resource availability.

Tanzania—The Hadza Tribe

In the heart of East Africa, Tanzania shelters one of the world's oldest hunter-gatherer societies, the Hadza. The Hadza's diet pivots on what their semi-arid woodland habitat generously offers.

During the wet season, the Hadza thrive on abundant wild honey, which constitutes a remarkable portion of their diet. They have developed a unique symbiotic relationship with the Greater Honeyguide bird, which leads them to beehives in exchange for the leftover beeswax. This natural bounty has offered them an energetic, readily available resource for millennia.

When the dry season rolls around, and honey becomes scarce, the Hadza leans heavily on the tubers from the *Vigna frutescens* (wild sweet pea) plant and other flora. Remarkably resilient, these plants endure the harshest droughts, offering a consistent and vital food source. The Hadza's diet highlights their adaptive ways and exemplifies how resource availability profoundly influences cultural eating habits.

The Andes—The Aymara People

High up in the rugged terrains of the Andes, the Aymara people have thrived by bending the scarce resources to their will. Their principal crop, the potato, demonstrates an extraordinary example of culinary adaptation.

The region's punishing altitude, cold temperatures, and infertile soils pose formidable challenges to most crops. Yet, the potato stands resilient. The Aymara, ingenious as they are, have harnessed the potato's hardiness, cultivating numerous varieties across the Andean slopes.

Further displaying their adaptive culinary skills, they invented a unique preservation technique. They expose harvested potatoes to the freezing night temperatures and the solid daytime sun to create chuño—freeze-dried potatoes. Chuño can last years without refrigeration, providing a reliable food source during lean times.

Micronesia—The Yapese People

Sailing to the tropical islands of Micronesia; here, the Yapese people live in harmony with the Pacific Ocean's vast expanse, exploiting its resources to sustain their way of life.

The sea teems with an array of marine life, offering the Yapese a steady supply of fish, mollusks, and crustaceans. They have developed intricate fishing techniques that respect the ocean's ebb and flow, keeping the ecosystem balanced while securing their food supply. Their diet reflects the ocean's bounty, enriched with diverse seafood and seaweeds.

However, their island geography also shapes their diet in unique ways. On Yap Island, fertile soil is at a premium. It is not just land; it is a resource. The scarcity of arable land led the Yapese to develop taro, a robust root vegetable, as their primary crop. Taro is cultivated in carefully managed terraces and serves as a staple, providing a reliable source of carbohydrates.

To complement their diet, the Yapese also gather fruit and nuts from the lush tropical forests. Breadfruit and coconut, both naturally abundant and highly nutritious, hold a significant place in their meals. Thus, the Yapese people's cuisine beautifully mirrors the resources that their tropical island paradise provides.

Here are some other tribes in example:

- **Africa** - The San People of the Kalahari Desert
- **Asia** - The Sherpas of Nepal
- **Australia** - The Aboriginal People
- **Caribbean** - The Taino People of Puerto Rico
- **Europe** - The Sami People of Scandinavia
- **Japan** - The Ainu
- **Middle East** - The Bedouin Tribes of the Arabian Desert
- **North America** - The Inupiat People of Alaska
- **Oceania** - The Maori of New Zealand
- **South America** - The Quechua People of Peru

Despite their vast geographical and climatic differences, each of these cultures bears a common thread—a story of survival and adaptation. Their eating habits, molded by the resources available, reflect the remarkable human capacity to make the most of their environment.

Now that we have unpacked some global cultures, let us take a tour of our gut variations and how they influence our digestion.

Genetic Gut Variations and Their Impact on Digestion

Genetic gut variations profoundly influence the intricate process of digestion, unveiling the diversity of human biology in the landscape of food processing. Within the human population, many genetic differences shape how our bodies break down and absorb nutrients.

These variations affect the functioning of enzymes, the composition of gut bacteria, and the efficiency of metabolic processes. Consequently, individuals may experience differences in their ability to digest certain foods, tolerance to specific dietary components, and susceptibility to digestive disorders.

Exploring the impact of genetic gut variations opens doors to a deeper understanding of personalized nutrition and the intricate interplay between our genes and our digestive health.

Our gut microbiome, in our digestive tracts, plays an integral role in our overall health, influencing everything from our digestion to our mood and immune function. Scientific advancements have illuminated the intricate relationship between our genes and gut health, enabling us to understand how certain genetic gut variations can significantly impact digestion (Goodrich et al., 2017).

FUT2

First on our list is the FUT2 gene. This gene, which helps produce the "secretor status" protein, affects the bacteria that can survive and thrive in our gut. Non-secretors, or individuals with certain variations of the FUT2 gene, often exhibit a reduced diversity of gut bacteria. This lack of diversity can lead to inefficient digestion, increased susceptibility to certain gut infections, and a higher risk for conditions like IBD and celiac disease.

LCT

Then, there is the LCT gene, responsible for lactase production, the enzyme that breaks down lactose into simpler sugars. Many people worldwide experience a decrease in lactase activity due to a variation in this gene, leading to lactose intolerance. For these individuals, consuming lactose can result in symptoms like bloating, abdominal cramps, and diarrhea, indicating a digestive system in distress (Malik & Panuganti, 2019).

CYP1A2

We also have the CYP1A2 gene. It does not directly influence gut health but significantly impacts how our bodies metabolize certain substances, notably caffeine. Variations of this gene can slow down or speed up caffeine metabolism, affecting the balance of our gut microbiome. Overconsumption of caffeine for slow metabolizers can harm gut health and contribute to digestive issues such as acid reflux and stomach ulcers.

FADS 1-2

In addition, there is the FADS1/2 gene. Variations in these genes affect our ability to convert plant-based omega-3 and omega-6 fatty acids into active forms our bodies can use. People with certain variations of these genes might struggle with this conversion, potentially leading to an imbalance in the gut microbiome and associated digestive complications.

APOA5

Moreover, our bodies house the APOA5 gene, which is instrumental in triglyceride metabolism. Variants of this gene can lead to increased triglyceride levels, a form of fat in our blood. Researchers believe a direct relationship exists between these variants and a predisposition to non-alcoholic fatty liver disease (NAFLD), a condition often accompanied by gut dysbiosis, where the gut's microbial balance is disrupted, leading to poor digestion and other health complications (Safari & Gérard, 2019).

SHBG

Lastly, the SHBG gene, which influences sex hormone-binding globulin levels, plays a role in gut health. Alterations in this gene may lead to lower SHBG levels and, subsequently, an increased risk of metabolic syndrome characterized by insulin resistance. Researchers have linked metabolic syndrome to gut dysbiosis, suggesting a potential impact on digestion (Martinez et al., 2017).

All these genes paint a picture of our unique gut health landscape, demonstrating that our genetic makeup plays a critical role in dictating the state of our gut microbiome and, consequently, our digestive health. But it is also essential to remember that our lifestyle choices, like diet and exercise, significantly influence these outcomes. Although genetics can be seen as the proverbial loaded gun, it is often the environment that activates the trigger.

Future research in the field of nutrigenomics, the study of the interaction between diet and genes, promises to illuminate these intricate connections further. With this knowledge, we can strive towards personalized nutrition and health strategies designed to cater to our unique genetic gut variations and promote optimal digestive health. Understanding our gut's genetic predispositions brings us one step closer to a future where preventative health is not a one-size-fits-all approach but a tailored, individualized journey.

Next up, we unpack our "second brain."

Chapter 8:

The Gut as the "Second Brain"

Many of the gut signals reaching the brain will not only generate gut sensations, such as the fullness after a nice meal, nausea and discomfort, and feelings of well-being but will also trigger responses of the brain that sends back to the gut, generating distinct gut reactions. And the brain doesn't forget about these feelings either. Gut feelings are stored in vast databases in the brain, which can later be accessed when making decisions.
–Emeran Mayer

Our gut, intriguingly called the "second brain," holds a powerful sway over our bodies. Packed with countless neurons and neurotransmitters, it communicates directly with our primary brain, influencing mood, cognition, and overall health. This complex gut-brain dialogue is essential for our survival, processing crucial information from our environment through the foods we consume.

Understanding this "second brain" opens doors to improved well-being, innovative treatments for mental disorders, and a profound rethinking of what makes us truly human.

Let me dive straight into this chapter.

Gut-Brain Axis: Its Impact on Mental and Emotional Health

Dominating our internal ecosystem, the gut wields remarkable power over our mental and emotional well-being. This connection is so much more than a mere food processing hub; it is a critical commander, orchestrating numerous biological activities that directly influence our feelings and mental state.

As we delve deeper into this fascinating organ, we unravel its vast influence, uncovering its capability to impact mood, stress, and overall emotional balance. Recognizing the gut's command in these arenas reshapes our understanding of mental health and illuminates potential new treatment pathways.

The vast hemisphere of our emotional health intertwines with the bustling ecosystem within our guts. A compelling body of research emphasizes our gut's profound influence over our emotional well-being. Its silent command governs not just our physical health but also how we feel and respond to our environment emotionally (Clapp et al., 2017).

Indeed, our gut is a marvel of evolutionary design, teeming with trillions of microorganisms that carry out complex tasks that affect our moods and feelings. This dynamic microbial community (the gut microbiome) creates a powerful symbiosis with us, its host. Our gut microbiota consumes what we eat and metabolizes it into various byproducts, and those byproducts, in turn, can have a profound influence on our emotional well-being.

Take SCFAs, for instance. These molecules, produced by gut bacteria as they digest dietary fibers, carry out numerous roles, such as reducing inflammation and strengthening the gut barrier. More importantly, they communicate with the brain via the gut-brain axis, influencing our emotions. In fact, studies have shown that higher levels of SCFAs are associated with reduced anxiety and better mood (van de Wouw et al., 2018).

Gut bacteria can also produce neurotransmitters, chemicals that neurons use to communicate with each other. For instance, certain strains of Lactobacillus and Bifidobacterium can produce GABA, the brain's primary inhibitory neurotransmitter, which calms the nervous system and counteracts stress. Dysregulation in GABA signaling is a known factor in mood disorders like anxiety and depression.

Moreover, the gut microbiota influences the production of tryptophan, a type of amino acid that is a precursor to serotonin. As we know, serotonin regulates mood, and its imbalance is linked to several mood disorders. Hence, the gut's ability to regulate tryptophan levels directly impacts our emotional well-being (Cleveland Clinic, 2022).

Furthermore, recent discoveries have unearthed a novel communication route between the gut microbiota and the brain - the vagus nerve. This nerve serves as a major neural pathway in the gut-brain axis. It has been observed that gut bacteria can activate the vagus nerve, sending signals to the brain that influence emotional processing.

In light of these findings, it becomes clear that the gut, with its microbial inhabitants and biochemical capabilities, holds an authoritative stance on our emotional health. It is a delicate balance, a ballet of biological processes, where a misstep can trigger emotional turbulence. Recognizing and harnessing the power of the gut promises a new frontier in our quest for emotional balance and well-being. The knowledge that our gut is not merely a passive digestive organ, but an active participant in our emotional experiences, can shift our approach to mental wellness and the methods we employ to achieve it.

Emotional Health

Our gut houses millions of neurons and produces a vast range of neurotransmitters like the brain. One such neurotransmitter is serotonin, often labeled the 'feel-good hormone' due to its significant role in regulating mood, happiness, and anxiety. Fascinatingly, an estimated 90% of the body's serotonin resides in the gut. When our gut health thrives, serotonin production remains optimal, contributing to a positive emotional state. In contrast, disturbances in the gut, such as dysbiosis or inflammation, can disrupt serotonin production, leading to emotional imbalances and feelings of anxiety and sadness.

The gut microbiota plays an equally pivotal role in our emotional health. Emerging research suggests that a diverse and balanced gut microbiota can positively influence our emotional responses. For instance, certain strains of beneficial bacteria, often found in probiotic foods, have shown promise in reducing symptoms of anxiety and depression. These findings suggest that fostering a healthy gut microbiota might be a powerful, yet largely untapped, resource for managing our emotional health (Clapp et al., 2017).

Mental Well-Being

Moving from our emotional to mental health, the gut continues demonstrating its unyielding command. The gut-brain axis, a two-way communication system linking our central and enteric nervous systems, forms the epicenter of this influence. The messages relayed along this axis can shape our cognitive function, thought processes, and susceptibility to various mental health disorders.

Prominently, dysregulation in the gut-brain axis has been implicated in neurodegenerative diseases, such as Alzheimer's. Patients with these conditions often exhibit altered gut microbiota and increased gut inflammation, suggesting a possible gut-origin hypothesis for these diseases. Additionally, our 'second brain' influences our cognitive abilities, like memory and learning. Studies in mice have revealed that those with a healthier gut microbiota perform better in memory tests than those with an imbalanced gut (Clapp et al., 2017).

Moreover, the gut's potential role in mood disorders, including depression and anxiety, has become a recent research focus. An imbalance in gut microbiota can trigger an inflammatory response, causing the immune system to activate and produce cytokines. These immune system messengers can cross the blood-brain barrier and induce a state of "neuroinflammation," which research has closely linked to the development of depression. Therefore, maintaining gut health becomes crucial for our physical well-being and a balanced mental state.

The burgeoning field of psychobiotics, which confer mental health benefits, offers promising implications for mental health interventions. Certain strains of bacteria, such as *Bifidobacterium* and *Lactobacillus*, have demonstrated potential to reduce symptoms of depression and anxiety, underscoring the therapeutic potential of targeting the gut microbiota to treat mental health disorders (Zhu et al., 2022)

To conclude, the gut, the "second brain," has a commanding influence over our emotional and mental health. It is a pivotal player in the orchestra of our well-being, capable of shaping our mood, emotions, cognitive functions, and mental health. The burgeoning understanding of this influence ushers in an exciting era in healthcare, where innovative treatments for emotional and mental disorders might come from tending to our gut health.

It is a reminder that taking care of our gut goes beyond physical well-being; it is an act of nourishment for the mind and soul as well.

Next up is the gut's influence on depression and anxiety levels.

Gut Health's Influence on Anxiety and Depression

The gut's health plays a vital role in how we experience the world emotionally, underlining its extraordinary authority over our psychological well-being. Far from just a digestion machine, the gut wields considerable power in governing our emotions, particularly anxiety and depression.

As the commander of this biological orchestra, the gut can transmit signals that can alter our mood, contributing to or even instigating these mental health conditions. Grasping the might of the gut over our emotional state, we can explore new avenues for addressing psychological challenges like anxiety and depression.

The far-reaching influence of gut health significantly extends into mental health, particularly concerning disorders like depression and anxiety. Let us delve first into the complex dance between gut health and depression.

Depression

This pervasive mental health issue can profoundly impact an individual's quality of life. A growing body of research has begun to illuminate a potential relationship between compromised gut health and the onset and progression of depression (Schnorr & Bachner, 2016).

This gut microbiome can be compromised in various ways—poor dietary habits, lack of exercise, chronic stress, or antibiotic overuse. A compromised gut, marked by low diversity or an imbalance of gut bacteria, can disrupt this communication network. This disruption can lead to low-grade inflammation, a condition linked to depression. Additionally, an unhealthy gut can impair the production and regulation of mood-related neurotransmitters like serotonin, where 90% of our body's supply resides.

Several solutions can help address these issues. A foremost recommendation is dietary changes. Adopting a fiber-rich diet, fermented foods, and diverse plant-based foods can foster a healthier gut microbiome. Foods such as legumes, whole grains, fruits, vegetables, yogurt, and kefir are excellent sources. Similarly, limiting the intake of processed foods, high in sugar and unhealthy fats, can reduce inflammation.

Supplementation with probiotics and prebiotics can also promote gut health. Probiotics are good bacteria that can restore balance in the gut microbiota, while prebiotics serve as food for these helpful microbes. Regular exercise like cardio or weight lifting and stress management techniques like breathing or stretching can also support a healthy gut environment (Clapp et al., 2017).

Anxiety

Switching gears to anxiety, our gut wields a similar level of influence. Anxiety disorders are identified by persistent and excessive worry; an imbalanced gut microbiota can exacerbate these symptoms. Individuals with anxiety disorders often have a distinct gut microbiota composition compared to those without, suggesting a potential role of the gut in these conditions.

Like depression, a compromised gut can create problems by disrupting the delicate balance of neurotransmitters like GABA and serotonin, leading to heightened anxiety levels. Moreover, an unhealthy gut can trigger an inflammatory response, activating the immune system. This immune response can lead to increased production of cytokines, some of which can exacerbate anxiety symptoms.

Addressing gut health to manage anxiety involves strategies similar to those employed for depression. A nutrient-dense diet is paramount. Fruits, vegetables, whole grains, legumes, lean proteins, and fermented foods can support a balanced gut microbiota and reduce inflammation. Reducing the consumption of sugary and processed foods can help manage blood sugar levels, reducing anxiety symptoms.

Supplementation with probiotics and prebiotics may also be beneficial. Certain strains of probiotics, such as Lactobacillus and Bifidobacterium, have shown promise in reducing anxiety symptoms. Regular physical activities can help decrease stress levels, promote gut motility, and support healthy gut microbiota.

There are a range of mindfulness-based stress relieving techniques and cognitive-behavioral therapies that can be deployed. These methods can help individuals manage stress and anxiety, which can, in turn, support gut health.

In conclusion, the burgeoning field of gut-brain axis research reveals compelling links between gut health and mental health disorders like depression and anxiety. This expanding knowledge presents promising opportunities for novel treatment strategies. By nurturing our gut health, we can make strides toward managing and mitigating the profound impacts of these conditions, illuminating a path to better mental health through the power of the gut.

Now that we have unpacked the problems, let us look at some solutions for lifestyle and dietary changes to promote good brain-gut connection (Clapp et al., 2017).

Diet and Lifestyle Tactics for Enhanced Brain-Gut Interaction

Harnessing the influential power of the gut, we can utilize diet and lifestyle changes to optimize the vital brain-gut interaction, enhancing our overall well-being. The gut, a formidable commander in our bodily functions, can be guided through specific choices in our food and daily habits.

These tactics fortify our gut health and improve communication with the brain, shaping our emotions and mental clarity. Exploring and adopting these strategic changes opens the door to heightened health and improved management of our body's intricate systems.

Lifestyle Tactics

Lifestyle adjustments, focusing on physical exercise and mindfulness practices, can significantly enhance gut-brain interaction. Let us explore how.

Firstly, regular physical activity stands out as an influential factor. Exercise stimulates the production of certain brain chemicals, like serotonin and dopamine, which elevate mood. Moreover, it supports the growth of diverse gut microbiota. Researchers have found that individuals who engage in regular physical activity have more varied gut bacteria than their sedentary counterparts, a trait often associated with better health. Integrating a moderate exercise routine, such as brisk walking, swimming, or cycling, can enhance this essential communication line between the gut and the brain.

Secondly, stress management practices form a crucial component of this lifestyle adjustment. Chronic stress can negatively impact the gut microbiota and trigger inflammation, disrupting the gut-brain axis. Mindfulness-based stress reduction techniques like art therapy, nature walk, or static stretching. Not only can it help manage stress and foster a healthy gut-brain relationship, but it also reduces inflammation, enhances the gut's barrier function and promotes the diversity of the gut microbiota.

Furthermore, adequate sleep contributes significantly to this dialogue. Sleep deprivation can change the gut microbiota composition and disrupt the gut-brain axis, leading to issues like mood disorders and cognitive decline. Therefore, prioritizing good sleep hygiene can foster more robust gut-brain communication (Cataldi et al., 2022).

Dietary Tactics

Moving on to dietary strategies, what we eat plays a monumental role in dictating the health of our gut and, subsequently, the effectiveness of gut-brain communication.

The modern Western diet, heavy in processed, high-sugar, and high-fat foods, can wreak havoc on the gut microbiota and lead to inflammation, severely impairing the gut-brain axis. These foods should be limited. Conversely, a balanced diet with diverse, nutrient-dense, and fiber-rich foods can support healthy and diverse gut microbiota.

Whole foods like grains, vegetables, fruits, and lean proteins provide the nutrients necessary for a healthy gut. They are also rich in dietary fiber, which the gut bacteria ferment into short-chain fatty acids, potent compounds known to communicate with the brain and support the gut barrier.

Moreover, fermented foods, such as yogurt, kefir, sauerkraut, and kimchi, can provide probiotics, beneficial bacteria that can enhance the gut microbiota and positively influence the gut-brain axis.

In addition to these dietary changes, mindful eating can be instrumental in fostering a healthy gut-brain connection. This involves eating slowly, paying attention to the taste and texture of food, listening to hunger and fullness cues, and minimizing distractions during meals.

Mindful eating can help curb overeating and promote better digestion. It encourages a more thoughtful approach to food choices, favoring foods nourishing gut microbiota and strengthening the gut-brain axis. Cooking tactics, too, can aid in this process. Preparing meals from scratch, using fresh, unprocessed ingredients, can enhance the nutritional quality of food and support gut health.

In conclusion, the power to enhance our gut-brain interaction lies significantly within our lifestyle and dietary choices. By integrating regular exercise, stress management techniques, mindful eating practices into our lives, and a balanced, nutrient-dense diet, we can foster a healthy and robust gut-brain dialogue. This, in turn, opens the door to improved mental and emotional health, underlining the adage that a healthy gut indeed contributes to a healthy mind.

I am sure you are as curious as to the blood type diet. In the next chapter, I will answer your questions.

Chapter 9:

Eating for Your Blood Type—Fact or Fiction?

The Blood Type Diet has made such a difference-not so much to my shape, but to how I feel and my energy levels. –Cheryl Cole

Let me now delve into the "eating for your blood type" trend. Is it a fact or fiction? We will examine scientific findings, scrutinize anecdotal evidence, and explore whether following a diet plan tailored to your blood type can genuinely impact your health.

I aim to provide comprehensive insights to help make informed decisions about nutritional well-being. Are you ready to debunk myths and uncover truths together?

The Theory of Eating According to Blood Type

Does our blood type influence our dietary needs and responses? We will sift through scientific research, trace its origins, and decipher the potential impact on our health. My mission is to empower you with credible, transparent knowledge to fuel your wellness journey. No stone will be left unturned in our goal of understanding this theory.

Understanding the Theory

Eating according to blood type, also known as the blood type diet, is a nutritional philosophy based on the premise that people with different blood types (A, B, AB, and O) respond differently to certain foods. The idea is that your blood type can guide your dietary choices and lifestyle habits for optimal health and even assist in disease prevention.

The Theory's Origins

The blood type diet theory was popularized by Dr. Peter D'Adamo, a naturopathic physician, in his 1996 book *Eat Right 4 Your Type*. D'Adamo argued that our ancestors had different nutritional needs based on their blood types, which evolved at different historical periods. For instance, he suggested that type-O, the oldest blood type, requires a high-protein diet, while type-A, which emerged during agrarian times, is better suited to a vegetarian diet (Leech, 2017).

Trend Emergence

The blood type diet quickly became a trend in the late 1990s and early 2000s due to its novelty and simplicity. It was embraced by those seeking personalized dietary advice. D'Adamo's book sold millions of copies worldwide, contributing to the diet's popularity. Celebrities, including Cheryl Cole and Cliff Richard, reportedly followed the diet, bolstering its fame and allure (Integrated Health, 2012).

Busting Some Myths

Despite the diet's popularity, scientific support for the blood type diet theory is scant. Research studies examining the efficacy of the diet often produce inconclusive results. A systematic review in the National Library of Medicine in 2013 found no evidence to support the blood type diet's claims (Cusack et al., 2013).

In 2014, a large study published in Medical News Today debunked D'Adamo's theory. The researchers found no evidence to support the diet's core premise—that certain blood types are incompatible with specific food groups. Instead, they found that adherence to particular diets—such as those recommended for blood type-A or O—could be beneficial. Still, the benefits were unrelated to an individual's blood type (Ellis, 2014).

In 2019, another review article in the National Library of Medicine reaffirmed these findings, stating that no scientific evidence supports the claim that dietary requirements vary by blood type. The researchers concluded that following the diets recommended for any of the blood types could potentially result in health improvements due to a balanced diet, not because of blood type (Barnard et al., 2020).

So, while the theory of eating according to blood type presents an intriguing concept for personalized nutrition, it lacks robust scientific evidence to substantiate its claims. Healthy diets tend to share common traits like plenty of lean proteins, whole grains, fruits, and vegetables, regardless of blood type. Therefore, following dietary advice based on established nutritional science and personal health conditions is crucial, rather than focusing solely on blood type. As always, consider consulting with a healthcare provider or a dietitian for personalized advice.

Research and Concepts of the Blood Type Diet Theory

Now, we will investigate the scientific rationale, inspect the fundamental principles, and unearth the claims made by its proponents. Join me as we explore this unique diet paradigm and its implications for our health. Ready to sift fact from fiction and gain clarity about this dietary approach?

Key Concepts

Each blood type, according to D'Adamo, reflects the dietary patterns of our ancestors and possesses its unique traits:

1. **Type-O:** Considered the oldest blood type, D'Adamo recommends a high-protein diet rich in lean meats, poultry, fish, and limited grains and dairy. He suggests that these individuals respond well to intense physical exercise.
2. **Type-A:** Believed to emerge in agricultural societies, a vegetarian diet full of fruits, vegetables, grains, beans, legumes, nuts, and seeds suits this blood type best, as per D'Adamo. He advocates for gentle exercise for Type-A individuals.
3. **Type-B:** Allegedly developed among nomadic tribes, Type-B individuals purportedly have a tolerant digestive system that can handle most food groups except corn, wheat, tomatoes, peanuts, sesame seeds, and chicken. D'Adamo recommends moderate exercise for this group.
4. **Type-AB:** Supposedly the youngest and rarest, and a mix of A and B, this blood type supposedly does well with a diet that balances the type-A and B diets. Relaxation techniques and calming exercises work best for this group, according to D'Adamo.

More Scientific Research

While the blood type diet has attracted attention, the scientific validity of its claims remains questionable due to insufficient comprehensive research.

Although this enjoys a fair share of popularity, it is important to note that the broader scientific fraternity has raised concerns regarding its evidential basis.

A study published in 2020 in the National Library of Medicine researched the association between the ABO blood group and the incidence of heart disease and diabetes. They found that while the blood group was associated with the risk of these conditions, there was no indication that specific dietary practices influenced this risk, contradicting the blood type diet theory (Parente, 2020).

In a 2021 meta-analysis also in the National Library of Medicine, scientists investigated the impact of blood type diets on biomarkers of cardiometabolic health. They found that the improvements observed were not blood type-specific, suggesting that overall diet quality, rather than blood-type-tailored diets, was the driver of health benefits (Barnard, 2021).

Consequently, these studies suggest that the central tenets of the blood type diet—that one's blood type should dictate dietary practices for optimal health—may not hold water under the lens of rigorous scientific examination.

Practical Considerations for Personalized Nutrition

This section will illuminate practical considerations for tailoring nutrition to your unique needs. From interpreting genetic tests to leveraging lifestyle data and bridging nutrient gaps, our discussion will provide actionable insights for your wellness voyage.

The Basis of Personalized Nutrition

Personalized nutrition represents a novel approach to health and wellness, striving to tailor dietary recommendations to individual biological and lifestyle factors. One such factor is blood type, a concept popularized by the blood type diet. However, while the idea seems attractive, it is crucial to consider its practical aspects and scientific validity.

Consider the Science

As we have previously discussed, this diet needs more substantial scientific backing. Research studies, such as those mentioned in the previous section, found no significant correlation between blood type-specific diets and the proposed health benefits. Hence, it is pivotal to base decisions on well-researched and scientifically validated factors while considering personalized nutrition.

Factor in Your Individual Health Status

Your health status, including any chronic conditions or metabolic imbalances, should precede blood type when determining a diet plan. Tailoring a diet to manage specific health conditions is often more beneficial. For instance, someone with diabetes would find it more helpful to follow a diet focused on blood sugar control rather than a generalized diet for their blood type.

Take Into Account Preferences and Lifestyle

A successful diet fits seamlessly into your lifestyle and considers your food preferences. If a diet is too restrictive or does not align with your routine and preferences, it becomes challenging to maintain long-term. For instance, a type-O vegetarian individual might struggle with the meat-heavy diet that this diet prescribes.

Consult a Medical Professional

While adopting diet trends like the blood type diet is tempting, it is essential to consult a medical practitioner before making any significant dietary changes. They can provide personalized advice based on a comprehensive understanding of your health history and current status.

Broaden Your Scope of Personalization

Instead of focusing narrowly on blood type, consider other genetic factors and biomarkers that have a more established link with nutrition. Genetic variants related to lactose intolerance, gluten sensitivity, and predisposition to specific nutrient deficiencies are far more influential on a diet than blood type.

Use Technology to Your Advantage

Technology has a significant role in personalized nutrition. Wearable devices can track physical activity, sleep patterns, and even heart rate variability, providing valuable insights for personalizing your diet and lifestyle habits.

Moreover, several apps and online platforms offer personalized diet plans based on a more comprehensive analysis of lifestyle, food preferences, and health status instead of relying on a single factor like blood type.

Always Refer Back to the Fundamentals of Healthy Eating

Regardless of blood type, some universal principles of healthy eating apply to everyone. These include consuming fruits and vegetables, prioritizing whole grains, choosing lean proteins, limiting added sugars and processed foods, and staying well-hydrated.

In pursuing personalized nutrition, it is crucial to critically evaluate and consider the practical implications of dietary theories like this diet. While personalizing nutrition can undoubtedly be beneficial, it is vital to base such personalization on scientifically validated factors, holistic understanding of one's health status, lifestyle, and food preferences.

Most importantly, remember that personalization should not compromise the universally accepted principles of healthy eating. Consulting with healthcare professionals ensures that your personalized nutrition approach is safe and effective.

Precautions and Alternatives of the Controversial Diet

Let us delve further into the much-debated blood type diet, highlighting potential precautions and exploring viable alternatives. We will question its credibility, inspect the potential pitfalls, and examine if it is the right approach for everyone. If it is not, fear not! We will unveil other proven and personalized nutritional strategies to lead you to wellness.

The Precautions

While the concept has gained popularity, there are crucial precautions to consider.

1. ***Lack of Scientific Evidence:*** From what we have already discussed, Rigorous scientific studies, such as those listed in the first section, have found no substantial evidence supporting this diet. Therefore, following this diet without scientific endorsement may not yield the promised benefits.

2. ***Potential Nutritional Deficiencies:*** Each blood type diet eliminates certain food groups, potentially leading to nutritional deficiencies. For instance, the type-O diet suggests limiting carbohydrate intake, which could lead

to insufficient fiber intake, which is crucial for gut health and disease prevention.

3. ***Overemphasis on a Single Factor:*** The diet assumes that blood type is the primary determinant of nutritional needs, overlooking other critical factors like age, gender, health status, and physical activity.

Exploring Suitable Alternatives

Considering these precautions, exploring other science-backed diet alternatives that offer personalized nutrition and promote gut health is wise.

1. **Mediterranean Diet:** This diet focuses on whole foods, including fruits, vegetables, whole grains, legumes, lean proteins, and healthy fats. We have already explored research showing its gut health benefits, such as decreasing the chances of heart disease and other chronic conditions. Its adaptability makes it an excellent alternative for a wide range of individuals.
2. **DASH Diet:** Developed to lower blood pressure, DASH emphasizes fruits, vegetables, lean proteins, and whole grains. It is flexible, promotes gut health, and is proven to help manage and prevent several chronic diseases.
3. **Intermittent Fasting:** Although not a diet per se, this eating pattern alternates periods of eating and fasting. It can cause weight loss and improved metabolic health and has been linked to better gut health by promoting diversity in the gut microbiome.

Below is a quick comparison table:

	Mediterranean Diet	DASH Diet	Intermittent Fasting
Flexibility	High	High	Moderate
Focus	Whole foods, balanced nutrients	Lowering blood pressure, balanced nutrients	Timing of meals
Gut Health Impact	High fiber intake promotes gut health	Balanced nutrients support overall gut health	May enhance gut microbiome diversity

While the blood type diet theory is compelling, it is essential to consider the potential precautions and the lack of scientific evidence supporting its principles. Thankfully, several viable alternatives can provide personalized nutrition and promote gut health.

These alternatives, including the Mediterranean diet, DASH diet, and intermittent fasting, are backed by scientific research and focus on balance and variety. As with any significant dietary change, it is essential to consult with a GP or dietitian to make the best decision for your individual health needs.

Pros and Cons of the Blood Type Diet

Now we will unmask its strengths and potential drawbacks. Does this eating regimen hold water scientifically? How does it fare in promoting a balanced, healthful lifestyle?

We will investigate these questions and more, taking a balanced look at this diet's merits and demerits. Our in-depth analysis will equip you to make informed decisions about your nutritional health.

Known Demerits

1. **Potential Nutrient Deficiencies:** Each blood type diet restricts certain food groups, potentially leading to nutrient deficiencies. For example, the Type-A diet recommends a vegetarian lifestyle, which, if not adequately planned, can result in inadequate intake of essential nutrients like vitamin B12 and iron, vital for gut health and overall well-being.
2. **Risk of Neglecting Individual Dietary Needs:** The blood type diet adopts a broad-stroke strategy that doesn't account for specific dietary requirements. This oversight could harm digestive wellness and overall health.
3. **Restrictive and Challenging to Follow:** This diet can be overly restrictive, making it challenging for some people to follow. This restrictiveness can negatively impact gut health, as a diverse diet helps foster a diverse gut microbiome, which is beneficial for health.
4. **Undue Stress and Psychological Pressure:** Another critical drawback of this diet is the potential for unnecessary stress and psychological pressure it may exert on its followers. This diet mandates strict

adherence to certain food choices based on one's blood type, which can lead to anxiety around meal planning and eating. This kind of dietary stress is not conducive to overall well-being, and it is also known that prolonged stress can negatively impact gut health by altering the gut microbiota balance. Therefore, with its rigid guidelines, the blood type diet could potentially exacerbate stress levels and consequently affect gut health.

Potential Merits

Despite these considerable concerns, this diet is not without its possible advantages.

1. **Promotes Awareness of Personalized Nutrition:** Although the blood type diet's scientific validity is contentious, it fosters awareness of personalized nutrition, which is a valuable concept. Understanding that individual dietary needs can vary is a step toward promoting optimal gut health and overall wellness.

2. **Encourages Whole Foods Consumption:** Each blood type plan emphasizes whole foods over processed ones. This focus benefits gut health, as whole foods, mainly fruits, vegetables, and whole grains, are fiber-rich and support a healthy gut microbiome.

3. **May Eliminate Problematic Foods for Some:** The diet's restrictions may inadvertently eliminate foods that cause issues for some individuals. For instance, if someone has undiagnosed gluten sensitivity, adhering to the type-O diet, which advises against wheat consumption, may improve gut health and overall well-being.

4. **Can Lead to Weight Loss:** Some individuals may experience weight loss on the Blood Type Diet due to its restriction, which could reduce calorie intake.

However, it is crucial to note that long-term weight loss and maintenance require sustainable dietary changes, not overly restrictive diets.

5. **May Trigger Healthier Habits:** For some, starting this diet might be the beginning of a healthier lifestyle journey. The emphasis on regular exercise, adequate hydration, and mindfulness in eating could positively influence gut health and overall health.

Up next, we look at gut health and balanced diets. Get ready to transform your entire lifestyle!

Chapter 10:

Balancing Diets and Gut Health

When diet is wrong, medicine is of no use. When diet is correct, medicine is of no need. –Ayurvedic proverb

In the quest for overall well-being, the importance of maintaining a balanced diet and nurturing a healthy gut cannot be overstated. The choices we make regarding our daily nutritional intake can profoundly impact our body's intricate ecosystem.

By embracing a holistic approach to eating, we empower ourselves to cultivate an environment conducive to optimal health. This section explores the complex connection between diets and gut health, shedding light on the interplay of nutrients and their influence on our digestive system.

From the fascinating world of probiotics to the role of fiber-rich foods, we delve into the science behind fostering a robust gut microbiome. Join me as I unravel the secrets to attaining a harmonious equilibrium within our bodies.

Strategies for Optimal Gut Health and a Balanced Diet

Achieving optimal gut health and maintaining a balanced diet are vital pillars of a vibrant and fulfilling life. The intricate relationship between our dietary choices and the well-being of our gut is of the utmost importance.

By embracing effective strategies, we can harness the power of nourishment to support a thriving digestive system. This enlightening section explores various techniques to promote gut health and achieve a harmonious dietary balance. From mindful eating practices to incorporating nutrient-rich foods, we embark on a journey to unlock the secrets of optimal well-being through the lens of our gut.

To unlock the transformative power of nourishment, it is essential to adopt effective strategies that support gut health and promote a harmonious dietary balance.

Adopt Global Diets Into Your Meal Plan

Exploring and incorporating traditional diets worldwide can offer valuable insights into promoting gut health and achieving a balanced diet. Traditional diets often emphasize whole foods, local ingredients, and culinary practices that have stood the test of time. By incorporating elements from Mediterranean, Japanese, Indian, or other traditional diets into a two-week meal plan, you can introduce a diverse range of flavors, nutrients, and cooking techniques.

Diversify Your Plates

Variety is essential when it comes to a balanced diet. Aim to incorporate a wide range of the five food groups into your meals. Each food group offers a unique blend of vitamins, minerals, and phytonutrients contributing to overall health. By diversifying your plate, you maximize the nutrient intake and support the body's diverse needs.

Embrace Fiber-Rich Foods

Incorporating various fiber-rich foods into our diets is a cornerstone for promoting gut health. Fiber acts as a prebiotic, fueling the growth of beneficial bacteria in the gut. Vegetables, whole grains, legumes, and fruits, are excellent sources of fiber. These foods not only provide essential nutrients but also support regular bowel movements, aiding in the elimination of waste and toxins.

Keep Hydrated

Adequate hydration is essential for maintaining optimal gut health. Water plays a crucial role in digestion, helping to break down food and facilitate nutrient absorption. It also aids in waste movement through the digestive tract, preventing constipation. Try to drink a decent amount of water throughout the day, and consider incorporating herbal teas or infused water for added flavor and hydration benefits.

Manage Stress Levels

Chronic stress can adversely impact our gut health. The gut-brain connection is well-established, and stress can disrupt the balance of our gut microbiota, leading to digestive issues. Incorporate stress management techniques into your routine, such as regular exercise, meditation, deep breathing exercises, or engaging in hobbies that bring you joy. Prioritizing self-care and finding healthy stress outlets can support your mental well-being and gut health.

Practice Mindful Eating

In our fast-paced lives, rushing through meals without paying attention to our body's signals is easy. Practicing mindful eating involves slowing down, savoring each bite, and being fully present during mealtime. This allows us to connect with our body's hunger and fullness cues, aiding in portion control and preventing overeating. Mindful eating also encourages us to appreciate our food's taste, texture, and aroma, enhancing our overall dining experience.

Prioritize Probiotics

Probiotics are tiny living organisms that confer health benefits when consumed. Including probiotic-rich foods in our diet, such as yogurt, kefir, sauerkraut, and kimchi, can enhance the diversity of our gut microbiota. Additionally, probiotic supplements can be considered under the guidance of a healthcare professional.

Reduce Added Sugars and Processed Foods

Processed foods, including sugary snacks and beverages, can disrupt the delicate balance of our gut microbiota. These foods are often low in fiber and high in unhealthy fats, additives, and artificial sweeteners. Overconsumption of added sugars can also lead to inflammation and negatively impact gut health. Opt for whole, unprocessed foods whenever possible, and choose natural sources of sweetness, such as fresh fruits or a sprinkle of cinnamon.

Turn to Professional Advice

Everyone's nutritional needs and gut health are unique. If you have specific concerns or conditions, it is advisable to consult with a registered dietitian or medical practitioner. They can supply personalized recommendations based on your individual needs, medical history, and goals.

In conclusion, achieving optimal gut health and maintaining a balanced diet require mindful choices and consistent efforts. By embracing fiber-rich foods, prioritizing probiotics, practicing mindful eating, staying hydrated, diversifying our plate, reducing processed foods and added sugars, managing stress, and seeking professional guidance, we can nurture our gut microbiota, enhance digestion, and support overall well-being.

Remember, small changes can make a significant difference, so start incorporating these strategies into your lifestyle today and experience the transformative power of a healthy gut and a balanced diet.

Incorporating traditional global diets into a two-week meal plan can add a sense of adventure, nourish your body with a wide range of nutrients, and support optimal gut health. By embracing the wisdom of traditional cuisines worldwide, you can experience the joy of cultural diversity on your plate while reaping the benefits of a balanced and nourishing diet.

Incorporating Diverse Cultural Foods Into a Healthy Eating Plan

An enriching way to enhance a healthy eating plan is by embracing the myriad flavors of diverse cultural cuisines. From Latin America's vibrant spices to Southeast Asia's delicate herbs, the world offers a cornucopia of culinary treasures that nourish body and spirit.

Immerse yourself in Mexican cuisine's vibrant colors and bold flavors, explore Thai dishes' aromatic curries and stir-fries of Thai dishes, or savor the earthy pulses and grains of African fare. Incorporating diverse cultural foods into your meals invites a harmonious symphony of tastes and textures that transform your eating plan into a global culinary tapestry.

Introducing diverse cultural foods into your healthy eating plan can bring a burst of flavors, expand your culinary horizons, and provide a wealth of nutritional benefits. By incorporating a variety of global cuisines into your meals over two weeks, you can embark on a delectable gastronomic adventure that nourishes the body and satisfies the taste buds. Let me dive straight into practical strategies to infuse your eating plan with vibrant colors, aromatic spices, and unique global ingredients.

Discover Staples From Around the World

Each culture has its own set of staple foods that form the foundation of its cuisine. Incorporate these into your meals to experience the essence of a particular culture. For instance, swap usual rice with couscous or quinoa for a North African twist, substitute pasta with *soba* noodles (made from buckwheat flour) for a taste of Japan, or opt for plantains instead of potatoes for a Caribbean touch. These global staples offer a new perspective on familiar dishes and contribute to a diverse and well-rounded eating plan.

Embrace Meatless Mondays

Take a page from vegetarian-friendly cultures and dedicate one day of the week to enjoying meatless meals. Explore the rich vegetarian traditions of countries like India, where lentils, chickpeas, and vegetables take center stage in dishes like dal and curries. Embrace the plant-based protein sources, such as tofu and tempeh, prevalent in Southeast Asian cuisine. By incorporating meatless Mondays, you add diversity to your eating plan, promote sustainability, and explore new avenues of flavor.

Garner Inspiration from Ethnic Websites and Cookbooks

Explore the wealth of culinary knowledge in ethnic cookbooks and reputable websites dedicated to international cuisine. These resources provide detailed recipes, cooking techniques, and cultural insights to help recreate authentic dishes in your kitchen. The possibilities are endless, from traditional Mexican enchiladas to Korean bibimbap or Middle Eastern falafel. Select a few recipes from different cultures and plan your meals accordingly to immerse yourself in a global culinary experience.

Incorporate Street Food Delights

Street food often reflects a culture's culinary heritage, offering quick, flavorful, and affordable dishes. Research street food favorites from around the world and recreate them at home. From Mexican tacos to Vietnamese *banh mi* (baguette) or Greek souvlaki, these handheld delights bring the essence of a culture's street cuisine to your table. Experiment with homemade sauces, fresh herbs, and various toppings to customize the flavors and recreate an authentic street food experience.

Indulge in Theme Nights

Designate specific nights of the week as "theme nights," where you focus on a particular cuisine. It could be an Italian pasta night, an Indian curry night, or a Thai stir-fry night. Research traditional recipes, compile a shopping list, and prepare a complete meal that showcases the flavors, techniques, and presentation of that specific culture. Theme nights provide a cohesive dining experience and allow you to immerse yourself in the essence of a particular cuisine fully.

Open Your Mind to New Ingredients and Flavors

Leave the confines of your food comfort zone and explore the world of exotic spices, herbs, and ingredients. Experiment with the smoky flavors of paprika and cumin in Mediterranean cuisine, the tangy tamarind (legume) and turmeric in Indian dishes, or the zesty lime and lemongrass in Southeast Asian delicacies. Visit local ethnic grocery stores or explore online marketplaces to source authentic ingredients and spices.

Participate in Cultural Events and Food Festivals

Explore local communities for food festivals, cultural events, or ethnic restaurants that offer authentic dishes. These experiences provide opportunities to taste traditional foods prepared by native chefs and gain insights into different culinary traditions. Going to such events allows you to expand your knowledge of global cuisine, interact with culinary experts, and spark inspiration for incorporating new dishes into your healthy eating plan.

Share Your Experiences

Invite friends or family members to join this global gastronomic adventure. Organize potluck dinners where each participant prepares a dish from a specific culture, encouraging everyone to share their newfound recipes and experiences. This creates a sense of community and allows everyone to discover even more diverse dishes and traditions.

Tips for Optimal Digestion and Gut Microbiome Support

Nourishing your gut is not just about avoiding stomach upset—it is about establishing a healthy microbiome that fosters optimal digestion. This section delves into scientifically-backed strategies that supercharge gut health. You can expect practical tips, expert insights, and holistic approaches that align with your lifestyle.

I will teach you how to support your gut microbiome and transform your overall well-being. It is time to digest this information and lead a healthier, happier life. Get ready to embrace the world of gut health and unlock the secrets to better digestion.

Advice for Optimal Digestion

1. **Hydrate Well:** Begin your mornings with a cup of warm water and a dash of lemon. This simple habit kickstarts the digestive system and aids in flushing out toxins.
2. **Incorporate Fiber-Rich Foods:** Each meal should contain a good amount of fiber. Options like oats, lentils, apples, and broccoli help stimulate digestion and prevent constipation.
3. **Balance the Plate:** Follow the 50-25-25 rule. Half your plate should contain vegetables, one-quarter of complex carbs, and the remaining quarter with protein. This balance ensures a variety of nutrients, promoting better digestion.
4. **Portion Control:** Instead of three large meals, opt for five to six smaller meals throughout the day. This prevents overloading of the digestive system and ensures a steady release of energy.
5. **Mindful Eating:** Spend at least 20 minutes on each meal. Chew thoroughly and avoid distractions. This enhances nutrient absorption and reduces the risk of indigestion and bloating.
6. **Prebiotic and Probiotic Foods:** Include natural prebiotic foods like garlic, onions, and asparagus and probiotic foods like yogurt and sauerkraut. They support the growth of good gut bacteria and improve digestion.
7. **Avoid Late-Night Snacking:** Allow your digestive system to rest before bedtime. Aim for a 12-hour fast between dinner and breakfast.
8. **Limit Processed Foods and Sugars:** These can cause inflammation and disrupt the digestive process.

9. **Listen to your Body:** If certain foods consistently cause discomfort, consider getting tested for food intolerances.

Follow this plan for two weeks, noting any changes in your digestion or overall well-being. You might feel lighter, more energetic, and less bloated.

Gut Microbiome Guidance

1. **Diversify your Diet:** A varied diet leads to a diverse microbiome, which benefits gut health. Include various foods from the different food groups into your diet.
2. **Fermented Foods are Key:** Foods like kimchi, kefir, yogurt, and kombucha are rich in beneficial bacteria that can enhance gut microbiomes.
3. **Focus on Polyphenol-Rich Foods:** Polyphenols are plant compounds that stimulate healthy gut bacteria. Examples include green tea, dark chocolate, and olive oil.
4. **Stay Hydrated:** Water benefits the mucosal lining, helping good bacteria thrive.
5. **Exercise Regularly:** Physical activity can increase the diversity of gut bacteria. Aim for at least half an hour of moderate exercise most days.
6. **Quality Sleep:** Lack of sleep can negatively impact your gut microbiome. Strive for seven to nine hours of sleep per night.
7. **Consider a Probiotic Supplement:** Consider a high-quality supplement if you struggle to get enough probiotics from your diet. Consult with a healthcare provider to choose one that's right for you.
8. **Limit Antibiotics:** While necessary in some instances, excessive use of antibiotics can harm the gut bacteria.

Only use them under the supervision of a healthcare provider.

9. **Manage Stress:** Chronic stress can unbalance the gut microbiome. Exercises like deep breathing exercises, coloring therapy, and self-massage can help manage stress levels.
10. **Quit Smoking:** Smoking can harm the gut microbiota and lead to digestive issues.

Caring for your gut microbiome is a lifelong commitment, not a one-time effort. It requires healthy dietary habits, regular physical activity, stress management, and a balanced lifestyle. By embracing these habits, you invest in your long-term health and well-being.

Fiber's Role in Gut Health and Increasing Fiber Intake

Fiber is significant in maintaining gut health. It adds bulk to your diet, aiding digestion and promoting regular bowel movements. More importantly, fiber nourishes beneficial gut bacteria, bolstering the microbiome. To increase your fiber intake, include more vegetables, whole grains, fruits, and legumes in your meals. Gradually increase the intake and remember to drink plenty of water, as fiber works best when it absorbs fluid. Prioritize fiber for a healthy gut and improve overall well-being.

Fiber's Role in Gut Health

When it comes to maintaining the best gut health, the importance of dietary fiber cannot be overstated. Consuming ample fiber is instrumental in establishing a healthy and robust gut microbiome.

1. **Promotes Regular Bowel Movements:** Fiber adds bulk to the stool, aiding its passage through the digestive tract. This reduces the chances of constipation and promotes regular bowel movements.
2. **Feeds Beneficial Gut Bacteria:** Fiber is a primary food source for many beneficial bacteria in the gut. These bacteria convert fiber into short-chain fatty acids, which have numerous health benefits, including anti-inflammatory effects and strengthening the gut barrier.
3. **Supports Weight Management:** Fiber-rich foods tend to be more filling, helping to reduce excessive calorie consumption and aiding in weight management, which is beneficial for overall gut health.
4. **Prevents Digestive Conditions:** High-fiber diets can help prevent various digestive conditions, including diverticulitis, hemorrhoids, and GERD.
5. **Enhances Immune Function:** A fiber-fueled, healthy gut microbiome can bolster the immune system, as a significant part of the immune system resides in the gut.

Fiber is essential in nurturing a balanced gut ecosystem, promoting regular digestion, and maintaining overall gut health. However, it is important to note that not all fibers function similarly, and various fiber sources are recommended for optimal gut health.

Tips for Increasing Fiber Intake

Integrating more fiber into your diet does not mean discarding your culinary heritage. In fact, traditional diets across the globe abound with fiber-rich foods. Here is how to tap into these food traditions to boost fiber intake:

Mexican Cuisine: Mexico's culinary heritage offers a plethora of fiber-rich foods. Use black beans in tacos or burritos instead of meat for a fiber boost. Opt for whole-grain tortillas and incorporate more *nopal* (cactus), which is high in fiber, into salads and stews.

African Cuisine: Africa's diverse culinary landscape has plenty of fiber-rich options. Teff, a staple grain in Ethiopian and Eritrean cuisines, is high in fiber and can replace less nutritious grains. In West Africa, okra is a common vegetable often used in soups and stews and an excellent fiber source.

Middle Eastern Cuisine: This cuisine is known for its use of legumes, vegetables, and whole grains, all of which are rich in fiber. Opt for dishes like hummus, falafel, and tabbouleh, which feature chickpeas, lentils, bulgur, and various vegetables.

South American Cuisine: Quinoa, native to South America, is a complete protein and a great source of fiber. The black bean stew *(feijoada)* is fiber-packed in Brazil. And do not overlook the humble potato, native to Peru - especially the skin, which is particularly rich in fiber.

Scandinavian Cuisine: The Nordic diet is full of fiber-rich foods. Rye bread, a staple, is high in fiber. Berries, another common component, provide a sweet fiber source. Traditional dishes like *kåldolmar* (cabbage rolls) offer fiber-filled veggies, and root vegetables used in soups and stews also boost your fiber intake.

Southeast Asian Cuisine: Rice is a staple in this region. Switching to brown rice instantly increases fiber intake. Incorporating more local fruits, vegetables, and legumes, like jackfruit, yam, and mung beans, can also boost your meals' fiber.

When it comes to increasing fiber intake, it is a matter of making smart, conscious choices, no matter what your dietary traditions. Opt for whole grains, include more fruits, vegetables, and legumes in meals, and explore the fiber-rich aspects of culinary heritage. Incorporating these changes into your diet will boost fiber intake and contribute to a healthier, more balanced gut.

Two-Week Diverse Gut Health Eating Meal Plan

This two-week gut health meal plan brings together flavors from around the globe to nourish gut microbiomes. Packed with fiber, probiotics, and nutrient-dense foods, this plan offers an easy-to-follow roadmap for anyone seeking a balanced, diverse diet that supports gut health. So, enjoy tasty meals that nurture the gut and enhance overall wellness!

I have divided the 14 days into a daily theme to keep it fun and even included a shopping list. Here is your quick breakdown

1. **Day One:** Mediterranean
2. **Day Two:** African
3. **Day Three:** Japanese
4. **Day Four:** Inuit
5. **Day Five:** Indian
6. **Day Six:** Middle Eastern
7. **Day Seven:** Mexican
8. **Day Eight:** Iranian
9. **Day Nine:** Nordics
10. **Day Ten:** South American
11. **Day Eleven:** Thai
12. **Day Twelve:** Caribbean
13. **Day Thirteen:** Vietnamese
14. **Day Fourteen:** Latin American

Diet Day	Break-fast	AM Snack	Lunch	PM Snack	Dinner
One	Greek yogurt with honey, walnuts, and fresh berries	Handful of dried figs	Greek salad with feta and olives	Hummus with carrot sticks	Grilled fish with a side of tabbouleh
Two	Millet porridge with banana slices	Roasted chickpeas	Ethiopian lentil stew with teff injera	Orange slices	West African jollof rice with vegetables
Three	Miso soup with seaweed and tofu	Edamame	Sushi rolls with fresh vegetables	Seasoned nori strips	Grilled salmon with a side of fermented pickles
Four	Smoked salmon on whole grain toast	Frozen blueberries	Wild-caught fish stew with root vegetables	Handful of walnuts	Baked Arctic char with a side of seaweed salad

Diet Day	Break-fast	AM Snack	Lunch	PM Snack	Dinner
Five	Vegetable upma with coconut chutney	Roasted makhana (fox nuts)	Mixed vegetable curry with brown rice	Fresh mango slices	Dal with quinoa and side of fermented pickles
Six	Whole grain pita with labneh and za'atar	Handful of dates	Chickpea falafel with tahini sauce	Cucumber slices with tzatziki	Chicken shawarma with whole grain pita and pickles
Seven	Huevos rancheros with whole grain tortillas	Guacamole with jicama sticks	Veggie-filled black bean burrito	Sliced papaya	Grilled fish tacos with salsa and avocado
Eight	Whole grain bread with feta cheese and walnuts	Fresh cherries	Herb rice with grilled vegetables	Handful of pistachios	Ghormeh sabzi (Persian herb stew) with brown rice

Diet Day	Break-fast	AM Snack	Lunch	PM Snack	Dinner
Nine	Rye bread with smoked salmon and dill	Sliced apples	Nordic salad with root vegetables and herring	Handful of lingonberries	Baked cod with new potatoes and pickled cucumber
Ten	Quinoa porridge with berries	Sliced avocado	Quinoa salad with beans, corn, and	Handful of Brazil nuts	Grilled chicken with a side of black bean stew
Eleven	Rice congee with fermented tofu	Fresh mango slices	Green papaya salad with shrimp	Sliced guava	Thai red curry with vegetables and brown rice
Twelve	Tropical fruit smoothie with coconut milk	Handful of cashews	Jerk chicken with rice and peas	Fresh pineapple slices	Grilled fish with a side of callaloo

Diet Day	Break-fast	AM Snack	Lunch	PM Snack	Dinner
Thirteen	Pho with vegetables and tofu	Fresh lychee	Rice paper rolls with shrimp and herbs	Sliced dragon fruit	Lemongrass chicken with brown rice and pickled vegetables
Fourteen	Arepa with cheese and avocado	Sliced papaya	Ceviche with sweet potato and corn	Fresh guava slices	Pabellón criollo with black beans, plantains, and shredded beef

Shopping List

- Apples
- Arctic char (fish)
- *Arepa* (cornmeal cakes)
- Avocados
- Bananas
- Beans (black, lentil, chickpeas)
- Beef (shredded)
- Berries (blueberries, lingonberries, mixed berries)
- Brazil Nuts

- Brown Rice
- *Callaloo* (leaf vegetable stew)
- Cashews
- Cheese (feta)
- Cherries
- Chicken (breast, shredded)
- Chickpeas
- Coconut milk
- Cod
- Corn
- Cucumbers
- Dates
- Dill
- Dragon fruit
- *Edamame* (whole immature soybeans)
- Figs (dried)
- Fish (white fish for grilling, salmon)
- Fox nuts (*Makhana*)
- Guava
- Herring
- Honey
- Hummus
- *Injera* (a flat bread, resembling a pancake/crepe)

- *Jicama* (turnip/potato/yam bean)
- *Labneh* (yogurt cheese)
- Lemongrass
- Lychee
- Mango
- Millet (round, whole grains)
- New potatoes (young potatoes)
- Nori strips (slices of seaweed)
- Nuts (walnuts, pistachios)
- Olives
- Oranges
- Papayas
- Peas
- Pickles (fermented, cucumber)
- Pita bread (whole grain)
- Plantains (bananas)
- Quinoa
- Rice (sushi, basmati)
- Root vegetables (various for soups and salads)
- Rye bread
- Shrimp
- Smoked salmon
- *Tabouleh* (herb and bulgur salad)

- *Tahini* (sesame seed paste)
- Teff (similar to a poppy seed)
- *Tofu* (condensed soy milk) (firm, fermented)
- Tomatoes
- Walnuts
- Whole grain tortillas
- Yogurt (Greek, plain)

You are all set! Get ready for a two-week culinary adventure that your gut will love. Enjoy this deliciously diverse meal plan, filled with fiber-rich, nutrient-dense foods and probiotics, celebrating traditional diets worldwide!

How about some beverages to go with those meals? See the next section for inspiration.

Drinks Great for Gut Health

Keeping the gut healthy can be as simple as making mindful drink choices. Hydration is crucial for digestion and nutrient absorption; some beverages can even help nourish and balance the gut flora.

The right drinks can support a thriving gut ecosystem, from probiotic-rich options to soothing herbal infusions. So, when reaching for your next drink, remember that gut health is only a sip away!

A well-balanced diet is crucial for governing a healthy gut, and our drinks play an equally important role. Let us explore an array of both hot and cold beverages from around the world that can support gut health.

Water

The most straightforward and most crucial drink for gut health is water. It aids digestion, nutrient absorption, and maintaining a healthy mucosal lining in the gut. Staying well-hydrated can prevent constipation and ensure a smoothly running digestive system.

Probiotic Drinks

Probiotics are live bacteria that are good for gut health. Incorporating drinks rich in probiotics into your daily routine can improve digestive health and immunity.

1. **Amazake***:* A traditional sweet, low-alcohol Japanese beverage made from fermented rice. Packed with probiotics, Amazake helps promote a healthy gut microbiome.
2. **Kefir:** From the Caucasus Mountains, kefir is a fermented milk drink loaded with probiotics. It promotes better digestion and supports a balanced gut microbiome.

Herbal Teas

Several herbal teas are known for their digestive benefits and can soothe the gut.

1. **Peppermint Tea:** It can relieve digestive symptoms such as gas, bloating, and indigestion.
2. **Ginger Tea:** Consumed worldwide, ginger tea can help with nausea and gastric emptying.
3. **Fennel Tea:** Popular in India and the Middle East, fennel tea can relieve bloating and cramping.
4. **Chamomile Tea:** Known for its calming properties, it can also soothe an upset stomach and aid digestion.

Bone Broth

This savory elixir, enjoyed worldwide, is rich in collagen and glutamine, which can heal your gut lining and reduce intestinal inflammation.

Traditional Drinks

1. **Masala Chai:** A staple in India, masala chai is a spiced tea made with aromatic herbs and spices. Ginger and cardamom, key ingredients, are excellent for digestion.
2. **Switchel***:* This North American beverage, made from apple cider vinegar, ginger, and sweetener, can help balance stomach pH levels and improve digestion.
3. **Pulque***:* An ancient Mexican drink made from the fermented juice of the *maguey* (agave) plant, pulque is filled with probiotics.
4. **Tibicos (Water Kefir)**: Originating in Mexico, this fermented beverage from water kefir grains provides a fizzy, probiotic-packed drink.

Fruit and Vegetable Juices

Freshly squeezed fruit and vegetable juices provide a wealth of nutrients that can boost gut health.

1. **Pineapple Juice:** It contains bromelain, an enzyme that aids digestion.
2. **Beet Juice:** It can improve digestion by increasing the production of stomach acid.
3. **Cabbage Juice:** Known for its ulcer-healing abilities, it benefits gut health.

Fermented Dairy Drinks

1. **Ayran***:* A traditional drink in many Middle Eastern countries, ayran is a mixture of yogurt, water, and

sometimes a pinch of salt. It is a probiotic-rich beverage that supports gut health.

2. **Dooghː** A popular drink in Iran and neighboring countries, doogh is a fermented yogurt beverage often flavored with mint. Its probiotic content aids in maintaining a healthy gut ecosystem, offering digestive benefits and a refreshing taste.

Now doesn't this chapter just make the mouth water?

Gut to Glory:

Unleashing the Power Within for a Vibrant Life

Sorry, there's no magic bullet. You gotta eat healthily and live healthily to be healthy and look healthy—end of story. –Morgan Spurlock

Unlocking the gut's potential is the key to a vibrant life. You boost digestion, enhance immunity, and fuel overall well-being by prioritizing gut health. Incorporate fiber-rich foods, hydrate with gut-friendly beverages, and nurture a diverse gut microbiome.

Remember, every small change contributes to this robust internal ecosystem. By taking these steps, you are not just aiding your gut—you are embracing a lifestyle that radiates health from the inside out.

The journey from gut to glory is a testament to the profound link between the gut and vibrant health. Take the reins and unleash the power within!

Summary of Key Points

We delved into the fascinating relationship between traditional foods and their profound effects on our gut microbiome. Here, we shed light on the pivotal role that dietary diversity plays in promoting a healthy gut.

We also embarked on a journey to understand the intricate workings of the gut microbiome. It is a vibrant community of microorganisms that resides within our digestive system and significantly influences our overall well-being.

Culture and diversity are essential themes that permeate this exploration. Traditional foods embody the richness of various communities and their unique culinary practices. They are a tribute to the diverse array of ingredients, flavors, and preparation methods that have evolved over generations.

The profound link between our gut and brain, known as the gut-brain axis, is another crucial aspect we examined. We discovered how traditional foods can positively impact our mental well-being, recognizing the importance of dietary factors in nurturing a healthy mind.

Traditional foods emerge as champions in the realm of gut health. They offer a treasure trove of dietary fiber, probiotics, and prebiotics, all of which contribute to the flourishing of our gut microbial diversity and optimal digestion.

While contrasting traditional diets with the modern ones prevalent today, we uncovered the detrimental effects of highly processed foods and the decline of dietary diversity on our gut microbiota. This exploration ignited a call to rekindle our appreciation for traditional foods and their potential to restore balance and vitality to our digestive systems.

Drawing from real-life case studies, we showcased the tangible impact of traditional diets on gut health. We uncovered the profound conventional food influence practices on overall well-being by examining specific cultural communities and their remarkable health outcomes.

In our quest to bridge the gap between tradition and modernity, we offered practical strategies for incorporating traditional foods into our daily lives. Lastly, we guided sourcing authentic ingredients, adapting traditional recipes to suit modern tastes, and fostering cultural diversity through our food choices.

Final Thoughts on Gut Health and Traditional Diets

Understanding the intricate link between gut health and overall well-being has been rewarding. Traditional diets' decisive role in nurturing our gut should be noticed. Each cuisine, from Mexico to Scandinavia, Africa to Asia, offers a wealth of fiber-rich, fermented, and probiotic foods that naturally nourish our gut. This universal connection to our ancestors and cultural heritage exemplifies food's power as medicine.

Embracing traditional diets means preserving culinary heritage and upholding the wisdom of centuries-old eating practices. These practices naturally support a thriving gut microbiome, demonstrating a symbiotic relationship between nature, our bodies, and health. With every sip of a fermented drink and every bite of a fiber-rich meal, we make conscious choices that uphold this relationship and foster better health.

The journey to gut health does not demand drastic changes; instead, a return to our roots, respecting the wisdom inherent in traditional diets. This is a gentle reminder that the path forward sometimes involves looking back. Here is to a healthier gut and a healthier you, naturally sustained by the rich tapestry of global food traditions.

Future Directions on Gut Health Research

As we look toward the future of gut health, the exciting possibilities are endless. The human microbiome, once an underexplored field, is now literally at the forefront of health and wellness research. Scientists are delving deeper into understanding the intricate web of microorganisms in our gut, uncovering their vast influence on our overall health.

Emerging research shows that gut health is not just about digestion. It is about mind-body connection, immunity, disease prevention, and mood regulation. As we advance our understanding, we realize that maintaining gut health could be pivotal in managing complex conditions, from mental health disorders to autoimmune diseases.

In parallel, our understanding of diet's role in shaping the gut microbiome is deepening. The rise of personalized nutrition, leveraging individual genetic makeup and microbiome composition, is an exciting prospect. Imagine a world where diet recommendations are fine-tuned to your unique biology, optimizing gut health and, by extension, overall wellness.

Further, advancements in biotechnology are paving the way for more comprehensive and accessible gut health monitoring. Home-based microbiome testing kits and digital health platforms focused on gut health are growing trends allowing individuals to understand better and manage their gut health.

While the future holds many exciting prospects, the fundamentals of gut health remain the same. A balanced, diverse diet rich in fiber, hydration, stress management, and regular physical activity is critical to maintaining a healthy gut. These timeless principles and cutting-edge scientific understanding, and technology set the stage for a revolution in gut health management.

The road ahead in the realm of gut health is one of discovery, innovation, and potential. It is a journey that takes us deeper into ourselves, towards a future where health truly begins in the gut. As we venture into this exciting frontier, one thing is clear—taking care of our gut is caring for our future. With every new revelation and research breakthrough, we are not just learning about our microbiome; but the essence of being human.

Over to You!

The path forward in gut health holds exciting promises, with an emerging focus on the power of traditional diets. This is your opportunity to take charge and harness the power of time-honored culinary wisdom for a healthier gut.

Our journey through the realm of gut health has illuminated its profound impact on our overall well-being. Future research will undoubtedly delve deeper, uncovering more about our intricate internal ecosystem. Alongside, there is a resurgence of interest in ancient food wisdom, with science validating what our ancestors knew: traditional diets are rich in gut-friendly nutrients, making them a potent force for maintaining gut health.

This understanding provides us with powerful tools. The nourishing probiotic-rich ferments, the fiber-filled whole foods, and the nutrient-dense recipes passed down through generations are all keys to unlocking optimum gut health. Integrating traditional diets into everyday meal plans can transform your gut health, optimizing digestion, immunity, mental well-being, and overall health.

At the same time, we can look forward to innovations in biotechnology and personalized nutrition, making gut health management more precise and accessible. Imagine having tailored diet plans based on your unique gut microbiome or home-based testing kits that provide insights into gut health.

Yet, amidst these advancements, you hold the power to shape your health starting today. You have the knowledge, the insights, and the tools. You have the world's traditional diets at your fingertips. What remains is the action.

So, incorporate that sauerkraut into meals, enjoy that miso soup, sip on the kefir, or relish a serving of fiber-rich beans. With every meal, you have the opportunity to support gut health. The future of gut health is not just in labs and research papers, but in our kitchens, plates, and daily routines.

The journey to gut health is personal, steeped in the richness of global food traditions and the exciting prospects of scientific advancements. Embrace this journey, tap into the wisdom of traditional diets, and you will be empowering not just your gut but your holistic health. The future of gut health is here. The question is, are you ready to embrace it?

References

Albala, K. (2011). *Food cultures of the world encyclopedia. 2*, The Americas. Greenwood.

Albracht-Schulte, K., Islam, T., Johnson, P., & Moustaid-Moussa, N. (2020). *Systematic review of beef protein effects on gut microbiota: Implications for health. Advances in Nutrition: An International Review Journal.* https://doi.org/10.1093/advances/nmaa085

Alcock, J., Maley, C. C., & Aktipis, C. A. (2014). *Is eating behavior manipulated by the gastrointestinal microbiota? Evolutionary pressures and potential mechanisms.* BioEssays, 36(10), 940–949. https://doi.org/10.1002/bies.201400071

Alexander, H. (2019, November). 5 *benefits of a plant-based diet.* MD Anderson Cancer Center. https://www.mdanderson.org/publications/focused-on-health/5-benefits-of-a-plant-based-diet.h20-1592991.html

Allen, T. S., Bhatia, H. S., Wood, A. C., Momin, S. R., & Allison, M. A. (2022). *State-of-the-art review: Evidence on red meat consumption and hypertension outcomes.* American Journal of Hypertension, 35(8), 679–687. https://doi.org/10.1093/ajh/hpac064

Alternative protein sources: Balancing food innovation, sustainability, nutrition, and health: Proceedings of a workshop—in brief. (2022). In PubMed. National Academies Press (US). https://pubmed.ncbi.nlm.nih.gov/36548452/

Anderson-Haynes, S.-E. (2021, April 21). *Diet, disease, and the microbiome. Harvard Health* Publishing. https://www.health.harvard.edu/blog/diet-disease-and-the-microbiome-2021042122400

Aneli, S., Mezzavilla, M., Bortolini, E., Pirastu, N., Girotto, G., Spedicati, B., Berchialla, P., Gasparini, P., & Pagani, L. (2022). *Impact of cultural and genetic structure on food choices along the Silk Road.* Proceedings of the National Academy of Sciences, 119(47). https://doi.org/10.1073/pnas.2209311119

Aswell, S. (2018, January 29). *For a longer life and happier gut, eat more fiber.* healthline. https://www.healthline.com/health/food-nutrition/fiber-diet-good-for-gut-and-health

Authentic Mole sauce recipe. (2019). Allrecipes. https://www.allrecipes.com/recipe/223261/authentic-mole-sauce/

Aztec influences on modern Mexican cuisine. (2016, May 12). BENITOS Real Authentic Mexican Food. https://benitosmexican.com/mexican-food/aztec-influences-modern-mexican-cuisine/

Barnard, N. D., Rembert, E., Freeman, A., Bradshaw, M., Holubkov, R., & Kahleova, H. (2020). *Blood type is not associated with changes in cardiometabolic outcomes in response to a plant-based dietary intervention.* Journal of the Academy of Nutrition and Dietetics. https://doi.org/10.1016/j.jand.2020.08.079

Benefits of physical activity. (2021, November 1). Centers for Disease Control and Prevention; CDC. https://www.cdc.gov/physicalactivity/basics/pa-health/index.htm

Berg, J., & Jackson, C. (2021, May 12). *Nearly nine in ten Americans consume meat as part of their diet.* Ipsos. https://www.ipsos.com/en-us/news-polls/nearly-nine-ten-americans-consume-meat-part-their-diet

Berrazaga, I., Micard, V., Gueugneau, M., & Walrand, S. (2019). *The role of the anabolic properties of plant- versus animal-based protein sources in supporting muscle mass maintenance: A critical review.* Nutrients, 11(8), 1825. https://doi.org/10.3390/nu11081825

Bhatia, A. (2012, September 30). *Milk, meat and blood: how diet drives natural selection in the Maasai.* WIRED. https://www.wired.com/2012/09/milk-meat-and-blood-how-diet-drives-natural-selection-in-the-maasai/

Bian, X., Chi, L., Gao, B., Tu, P., Ru, H., & Lu, K. (2017). *The artificial sweetener acesulfame potassium affects the gut microbiome and body weight gain in CD-1 mice.* PLOS ONE, 12(6), e0178426. https://doi.org/10.1371/journal.pone.0178426

Biga, L. M., Dawson, S., Harwell, A., Hopkins, R., Kaufmann, J., LeMaster, M., Matern, P., Morrison-Graham, K., Quick, D., & Runyeon, J. (n.d.). *Overview of the digestive system.* Oregon State University. https://open.oregonstate.education/aandp/chapter/23-1-overview-of-the-digestive-system/

Bingham, A. (2016, January 28). *21 healthy Spanish recipes to make at home.* Spanish Sabores. https://spanishsabores.com/11-healthy-spanish-recipes/

Blazejczyk, A., & Kantor, L. (2018). *USDA ERS - Food availability and consumption.* Economic Research Service U.S. DEPARTMENT of AGRICULTURE. https://www.ers.usda.gov/data-products/ag-and-food-statistics-charting-the-essentials/food-availability-and-consumption/

Boonkerd, P. (2017, May 16). *Eating mindfully.* Awakenings, 13–14. https://issuu.com/sharontaylor47/docs/awakeningsmag_issue_14_webpdf

Cao, Y., Liu, H., Qin, N., Ren, X., Zhu, B., & Xia, X. (2020). *Impact of food additives on the composition and function of gut microbiota: A review.* Trends in Food Science & Technology, 99, 295–310. https://doi.org/10.1016/j.tifs.2020.03.006

Capritto, A. (2020, October 9). *12 scientifically proven benefits of the Mediterranean diet.* Verywellfit. https://www.verywellfit.com/health-benefits-of-the-mediterranean-diet-4842600

Cataldi, S., Poli, L., Şahin, F. N., Patti, A., Santacroce, L., Bianco, A., Greco, G., Ghinassi, B., Di Baldassarre, A., & Fischetti, F. (2022). *The effects of physical activity on the gut microbiota and the gut–brain axis in preclinical and human models: A narrative review.* Nutrients, 14(16), 3293. https://doi.org/10.3390/nu14163293

Celiac Disease - Symptoms and causes. (2021, August 10). MAYO CLINIC. https://www.mayoclinic.org/diseases-conditions/celiac-disease/symptoms-causes/syc-20352220

Chemical additives in highly processed foods destroy gut health, study finds. (2022, April 1). The Defender. https://childrenshealthdefense.org/defender/chemical-additives-processed-foods-gut-health/

Cheng, F. (2023, March 7). *The regional treasures of China and its rising popularity in Hong Kong.* Tatler Asia. https://www.tatlerasia.com/dining/food/the-rise-of-regional-chinese-cuisine-hong-kong

Cheryl Cole quote. (n.d.). AZ QUOTES. https://www.azquotes.com/quote/1416134

Chilton, S., Burton, J., & Reid, G. (2015). *Inclusion of fermented foods in food guides around the world.* Nutrients, 7(1), 390–404. https://doi.org/10.3390/nu7010390

Clapp, M., Aurora, N., Herrera, L., Bhatia, M., Wilen, E., & Wakefield, S. (2017). *Gut microbiota's effect on mental health: the gut-brain axis.* Clinics and Practice, 7(4). https://doi.org/10.4081/cp.2017.987

Clemente, Jose C., Ursell, Luke K., Parfrey, L., & Knight, R. (2012). *The impact of the gut microbiota on human health: An integrative view.* Cell, 148(6), 1258–1270. https://doi.org/10.1016/j.cell.2012.01.035

Cliff Richard and the blood type diet. (2012, June 28). Integrated Health. https://www.integratedhealth.com.au/cliff-richard-blood-type-die/#:~:text=Richards%2C%20who%20is%20blood%20type

Cohen, S. (2021, March 19). *If you want to boost immunity, look to the gut.* UCLA Health. https://www.uclahealth.org/news/want-to-boost-immunity-look-to-the-gut#:~:text=70%25%20of%20the%20immune%20system

Cohut, M. (2020, February 20). *Mediterranean diet linked to gut microbiome improvements.* MedicalNewsToday. https://www.medicalnewstoday.com/articles/mediterranean-diet-linked-to-gut-microbiome-improvements

Costa, M. A. de C., Vilela, D. L. de S., Fraiz, G. M., Lopes, I. L., Coelho, A. I. M., Castro, L. C. V., & Martin, J. G. P. (2021). *Effect of kombucha intake on the gut microbiota and obesity-related comorbidities: A systematic review.* Critical Reviews in Food Science and Nutrition, 1–16. https://doi.org/10.1080/10408398.2021.1995321

Culture and food traditions: By supporting healthy, diversified and culturally appropriate diets, agroecology contributes to food security and nutrition while maintaining the health of ecosystems. (n.d.). Food and Agriculture Organization of the United States. https://www.fao.org/agroecology/knowledge/10-elements/culture-food-traditions/en/

Cultures, food traditions and healthy eating. (2019). Canada's Food Guide. https://food-guide.canada.ca/en/healthy-eating-recommendations/enjoy-your-food/cultures-food-traditions-and-healthy-eating/

Cusack, L., De Buck, E., Compernolle, V., & Vandekerckhove, P. (2013). *Blood type diets lack supporting evidence: A systematic review.* The American Journal of Clinical Nutrition, 98(1), 99–104. https://doi.org/10.3945/ajcn.113.058693

de Vos, W. M., Tilg, H., Van Hul, M., & Cani, P. D. (2022). *Gut microbiome and health: Mechanistic insights.* Gut, 71(5), 1020–1032. https://doi.org/10.1136/gutjnl-2021-326789

Digestive system: Function, organs & anatomy. (2021, August 9). Cleveland Clinic. https://my.clevelandclinic.org/health/body/7041-digestive-system

Dimidi, E., Cox, S. R., Rossi, M., & Whelan, K. (2019). *Fermented foods: Definitions and characteristics, impact on the gut microbiota and effects on gastrointestinal health and disease.* Nutrients, 11(8), 1806. https://doi.org/10.3390/nu11081806

Ding, R., Goh, W.-R., Wu, R., Yue, X., Luo, X., Khine, W. W. T., Wu, J., & Lee, Y.-K. (2019). *Revisit gut microbiota and its impact on human health and disease.* Journal of Food and Drug Analysis, 27(3), 623–631. https://doi.org/10.1016/j.jfda.2018.12.012

Does your blood type impact your diet? (2023, January 21). Cleveland Clinic. https://health.clevelandclinic.org/blood-type-diet/

Ellis, E. (2021, February 8). *Global foods for a healthy plate.* Eat.right.org. https://www.eatright.org/food/cultural-cuisines-and-traditions/african/global-foods-for-a-healthy-plate

Ellis, M. (2014, January 20). *Popular blood type diet claims are "not valid," researchers find.* Medical News Today. https://www.medicalnewstoday.com/articles/271349

Eskimo diet recipes. (n.d.). Eat Smarter! https://eatsmarter.com/recipes/nutritional/diet/eskimo-diet

Farré, R., Fiorani, M., Abdu Rahiman, S., & Matteoli, G. (2020). *Intestinal permeability, inflammation and the role of nutrients.* Nutrients, 12(4). https://doi.org/10.3390/nu12041185

Flores, R. (2022, June 27). *10 gut healing drinks for improved gut health.* SUPRHMN. https://superhumn.com/gut-healing-drinks/

Floyd Jones, J. (2023, February 14). *12 foods to improve your gut health overnight.* EatingWell. https://www.eatingwell.com/article/8021156/foods-to-improve-gut-health-overnight/

Food additives. (2018, January 31). World Health Organization. https://www.who.int/news-room/fact-sheets/detail/food-additives

Forouhi, N. G., Krauss, R. M., Taubes, G., & Willett, W. (2018). *Dietary fat and cardiometabolic health: evidence, controversies, and consensus for guidance.* BMJ, 361, k2139. https://doi.org/10.1136/bmj.k2139

Gardiner, K. (2019, February 5). *Your shot photos show food culture around the world.* NATIONAL GEOGRAPHIC. https://www.nationalgeographic.com/travel/article/your-shot-photos-food-culture-around-world

Geiker, N. R. W., Bertram, H. C., Mejborn, H., Dragsted, L. O., Kristensen, L., Carrascal, J. R., Bügel, S., & Astrup, A. (2021). *Meat and human health—Current knowledge and research gaps.* Foods, 10(7), 1556. https://doi.org/10.3390/foods10071556

Godman, H. (2021, October 1). *Healthy gut, healthier aging.* Harvard Health Publishing. https://www.health.harvard.edu/staying-healthy/healthy-gut-healthier-aging

Goodrich, J. K., Davenport, E. R., Clark, A. G., & Ley, R. E. (2017). *The relationship between the human genome and microbiome comes into view.* Annual Review of Genetics, 51(1), 413–433. https://doi.org/10.1146/annurev-genet-110711-155532

Graham, R. (2022, December 21). *Why is eating meat bad for the environment and climate change.* Sentient Media. https://sentientmedia.org/why-is-eating-meat-bad-for-the-environment/

Gubbins, T. (2022, July 21). *Austin makes showing on list of top 20 vegan cities in U.S. - CultureMap Austin.* Culturemap AUSTIN. https://austin.culturemap.com/news/restaurants-bars/06-21-22-vegan-friendly-cities-new-york-austin-rebel-cheese/

Guglielmi, G. (2020, December 18). *How a vegetarian diet influences the gut microbiota.* MICROBIOMEPOST. https://microbiomepost.com/how-a-vegetarian-diet-influences-the-gut-microbiota/

Gut health quotes (22 quotes). (n.d.). Goodreads. https://www.goodreads.com/quotes/tag/gut-health#:~:text=The%20road%20to%20health%20is%20paved%20with%20good%20intestines

Hall, A. B., Tolonen, A. C., & Xavier, R. J. (2017). *Human genetic variation and the gut microbiome in disease.* Nature Reviews Genetics, 18(11), 690–699. https://doi.org/10.1038/nrg.2017.63

Hamburger. (2021, May 7). Wikipedia. https://en.wikipedia.org/wiki/Hamburger#:~:text=White%20Castle%20traces%20the%20origin

Hao, M. M., & Stamp, L. A. (2023). *The many means of conversation between the brain and the gut.* Nature Reviews Gastroenterology & Hepatology, 20(2), 73–74. https://doi.org/10.1038/s41575-022-00725-4

Health benefits of sorghum. (2020, May 12). KANSAS FARM FOOD CONNECTION. https://kansasfarmfoodconnection.org/spotlights/health-benefits-of-sorghum#:~:text=Sorghum%20can%20also%20help%20with

Healthy Indian recipes. (n.d.). BBC Goodfood. Retrieved June 6, 2023, from https://www.bbcgoodfood.com/recipes/collection/healthy-indian-recipes

Hemler, E. C., & Hu, F. B. (2019). *Plant-based diets for personal, population, and planetary health. Advances in Nutrition,* 10(Supplement_4), S275–S283. https://doi.org/10.1093/advances/nmy117

Hiskey, M. (2021, March 24). *As fermented foods rise in popularity, here's what experts say.* American Heart Association. https://www.heart.org/en/news/2021/03/24/as-fermented-foods-rise-in-popularity-heres-what-experts-say

Hoover, A. (n.d.). *Apple cider vinegar myths & facts.* West Virginia University. https://extension.wvu.edu/food-health/cooking/apple-cider-vinegar-myths-facts

Horn, J., Mayer, D. E., Chen, S., & Mayer, E. A. (2022). *Role of diet and its effects on the gut microbiome in the pathophysiology of mental disorders.* Translational Psychiatry, 12(1), 1–13. https://doi.org/10.1038/s41398-022-01922-0

Hornbuckle, W. E., Simpson, K. W., & Tennant, B. C. (2008). *Gastrointestinal function. Clinical Biochemistry of Domestic Animals*, 413–457. https://doi.org/10.1016/B978-0-12-370491-7.00014-3

Horton, B. (2021, February 18). *7 drinks for better digestion.* EatingWell. https://www.eatingwell.com/article/7889310/drinks-for-better-digestion/

Hossein Akhondi, & Ross, A. B. (2019, November 27). *Gluten and associated medical problems. National Library of Information*; StatPearls Publishing. https://www.ncbi.nlm.nih.gov/books/NBK538505/

Hunter, C. (2021, May 6). *Embracing a plant-based diet.* StanfordReport. https://news.stanford.edu/report/2021/05/06/embracing-plant-based-diet/

Huzar, T. (2021, April 3). *Boosting fiber intake for 2 weeks alters the microbiome.* MedicalNewsToday. https://www.medicalnewstoday.com/articles/short-term-increase-in-fiber-alters-gut-microbiome

Igo, C. (2023, February 6). *Mediterranean diet for beginners: Health benefits, foods to eat and how it works.* CNET. https://www.cnet.com/health/nutrition/mediterranean-diet-for-beginners-health-benefits-foods-to-eat-and-how-it-works/

Ito, A. (n.d.). *Kaiseki: the zen and the art of food.* NAN BAN. https://www.nan-ban.com/en/chronicles/kaiseki-the-zen-and-the-art-of-food

Jardon, K. M., Canfora, E. E., Goossens, G. H., & Blaak, E. E. (2022). *Dietary macronutrients and the gut microbiome: a precision nutrition approach to improve cardiometabolic health.* Gut, gutjnl-2020-323715. https://doi.org/10.1136/gutjnl-2020-323715

Kim, M.-H., Yun, K. E., Kim, J., Park, E., Chang, Y., Ryu, S., Kim, H.-L., & Kim, H.-N. (2020). *Gut microbiota and metabolic health among overweight and obese individuals.* Scientific Reports, 10(1), 19417. https://doi.org/10.1038/s41598-020-76474-8

Kim, M.-S., Yang, H. J., Kim, S.-H., Lee, H. W., & Lee, M. S. (2018). *Effects of Kimchi on human health.* Medicine, 97(13), e0163. https://doi.org/10.1097/md.0000000000010163

Knowles-Dellner, S. (2023, January 5). *Top 10 foods to try in Sweden.* BBC Goodfood. https://www.bbcgoodfood.com/travel/europe/top-10-foods-try-sweden

Kumar, A., Jhilam Pramanik, Goyal, N., Chauhan, D., Nevin Sanlier, Dr. Bhupendra Prajapati, & Chaiyavat Chaiyasut. (2023). *Gut microbiota in anxiety and depression: Unveiling the relationships and management options.* Pharmaceuticals, 16(4), 565–565. https://doi.org/10.3390/ph16040565

Kumar, M., Tomar, M., Punia, S., Dhakane-Lad, J., Dhumal, S., Changan, S., Senapathy, M., Berwal, M. K., Sampathrajan, V., Sayed, A. A. S., Chandran, D., Pandiselvam, R., Rais, N., Mahato, D. K., Udikeri, S. S., Satankar, V., Anitha, T., Reetu, Radha, & Singh, S. (2022). *Plant-based proteins and their multifaceted industrial applications.* LWT, 154, 112620. https://doi.org/10.1016/j.lwt.2021.112620

La Forge, T. (2018, December 10). *6 herbs and spices to fire up your digestion.* healthline. https://www.healthline.com/health/digestive-health/herbs-spices-recipe#1

Landsverk, G. (2020, March 3). *What eating too much meat can do to your body, from dehydration to the "meat sweats."* Insider. https://www.insider.com/what-eating-too-much-meat-does-health-side-effects-2020-3

Leech, J. (2017, June 4). T*he blood type diet: An evidence-based review.* healthline. https://www.healthline.com/nutrition/the-blood-type-diet-review

Leeming, E. R., Johnson, A. J., Spector, T. D., & Le Roy, C. I. (2019). *Effect of diet on the gut microbiota: Rethinking intervention duration.* Nutrients, 11(12), 2862. https://doi.org/10.3390/nu11122862

Levy, J. (2023, April 20). *Should my blood type determine how I eat?* Dr. Axe. https://draxe.com/nutrition/blood-type-diet/

Liew, W.-P.-P., & Mohd-Redzwan, S. (2018). *Mycotoxin: Its impact on gut health and microbiota. Frontiers in Cellular and Infection Microbiology*, 8. https://doi.org/10.3389/fcimb.2018.00060

Lindberg, S. (2022, January 6). W*hy the Mediterranean diet is one of the healthiest ways to eat — and how to get started.* INSIDER. https://www.insider.com/guides/health/diet-nutrition/mediterranean-diet

Lionel Tiger Quote. (n.d.). AZ QUOTES. https://www.azquotes.com/quote/577884

Loscalzo, R. (2018, December 11). *10 spices to improve your digestion naturally — and help keep your gut happy.* FOOD REVOLUTION NETWORK. https://foodrevolution.org/blog/spices-for-digestion/

MacGill, M. (2018, June 26). *Gut microbiota: Definition, importance, and medical uses.* MedicalNewsToday. https://www.medicalnewstoday.com/articles/307998

Makki, K., Deehan, E. C., Walter, J., & Bäckhed, F. (2018). *The impact of dietary fiber on gut microbiota in host health and disease.* Cell Host & Microbe, 23(6), 705–715. https://doi.org/10.1016/j.chom.2018.05.012

Malik, T. F., & Panuganti, K. K. (2019, February 22). *Lactose intolerance.* National Library of Medicine; StatPearls Publishing. https://www.ncbi.nlm.nih.gov/books/NBK532285/

Markowitz, R. H. G., LaBella, A. L., Shi, M., Rokas, A., Capra, J. A., Ferguson, J. F., Mosley, J. D., & Bordenstein, S. R. (2022). *Microbiome-associated human genetic variants impact phenome-wide disease risk.* Proceedings of the National Academy of Sciences, 119(26). https://doi.org/10.1073/pnas.2200551119

Martinez, K. B., Leone, V., & Chang, E. B. (2017). *Western diets, gut dysbiosis, and metabolic diseases: Are they linked?* Gut Microbes, 8(2), 130–142. https://doi.org/10.1080/19490976.2016.1270811

Mayer, B. A. (2021, October 18). *What the five elements can teach you about your personality and health.* healthline. https://www.healthline.com/health/mind-body/what-are-the-five-elements

Meat eating link to inflammation, worse gut health and MS. (2022, January 28). THE UNIVERSITY of SYDNEY. https://www.sydney.edu.au/news-opinion/news/2022/01/28/meat-eating-linked-to-inflammation-worse-gut-health-and-ms.html

Mediterranean diet quotes. (n.d.). PICTUREQUOTES. http://www.picturequotes.com/mediterranean-diet-quotes

Melore, C. (2021, December 1). *Food additive in many processed foods alters gut health, may cause disease.* StudyFinds. https://studyfinds.org/food-additive-alters-gut-health/

Merra, G., Noce, A., Marrone, G., Cintoni, M., Tarsitano, M. G., Capacci, A., & De Lorenzo, A. (2021). *Influence of Mediterranean diet on human gut microbiota.* Nutrients, 13(1), 7. https://doi.org/10.3390/nu13010007

Mexican food culture through the ages. (n.d.). DE LA CALLE. https://www.delacalle.mx/blogs/news/mexican-culture-foods

Mexican food: A short history of its origins. (2022, March 17). ON the BORDER. https://ontheborder.com.au/mexican-food-a-short-history-of-its-origins/

Mikstas, C. (2021, November 4). *Mexican dishes to enjoy (and avoid).* WebMD. https://www.webmd.com/diet/ss/slideshow-mexican-food-health#:~:text=Order%20the%20grilled%20chicken%2C%20lean

Mitrokostas, S. (2019, February 9). *6 ways the Mediterranean diet can affect your digestion.* INSIDER. https://www.insider.com/mediterranean-diet-effects-on-digestion-2019-2

Monaco, E. (2019, May 7). *9 recipes to make you feel the hygge: Discovering true Danish food.* ORGANIC AUTHORITY. https://www.organicauthority.com/organic-food-recipes/discovering-danish-food-with-9-recipes-to-make-you-feel-the-hygge

Monterrosa, E. C., Frongillo, E. A., Drewnowski, A., de Pee, S., & Vandevijvere, S. (2020). *Sociocultural influences on food choices and implications for sustainable healthy diets.* Food and Nutrition Bulletin, 41(2), 59S73S. https://doi.org/10.1177/0379572120975874

Mudge, L. (2022, March 29). *What is gut health and why is it important?* LIVESCIENCE. https://www.livescience.com/what-is-gut-health-and-why-is-it-important

Naidoo, U. (2019, March 27). *Gut feelings: How food affects your mood.* Harvard Health Publishing; Harvard Medical School. https://www.health.harvard.edu/blog/gut-feelings-how-food-affects-your-mood-2018120715548

Narzary, Y., Das, S., Goyal, A. K., Lam, S. S., Sarma, H., & Sharma, D. (2021). *Fermented fish products in South and Southeast Asian cuisine: indigenous technology processes, nutrient composition, and cultural significance.* Journal of Ethnic Foods, 8(1). https://doi.org/10.1186/s42779-021-00109-0

Negrete-Romero, B., Valencia-Olivares, C., Baños-Dossetti, G. A., Pérez-Armendáriz, B., & Cardoso-Ugarte, G. A. (2021). *Nutritional contributions and health associations of traditional fermented foods.* Fermentation, 7(4), 289. https://doi.org/10.3390/fermentation7040289

9 facts on gut bacteria and mental health, probiotics and depression. (2020, July 3). Atlas Biomed. https://atlasbiomed.com/blog/9-ways-gut-bacteria-and-mental-health-probiotics-and-depression-are-linked/#:~:text=That

Nishijima, S., Suda, W., Oshima, K., Kim, S.-W., Hirose, Y., Morita, H., & Hattori, M. (2016). *The gut microbiome of healthy Japanese and its microbial and functional uniqueness. DNA Research: An International Journal for Rapid Publication of Reports on Genes and Genomes*, 23(2), 125–133. https://doi.org/10.1093/dnares/dsw002

Nova, E., Gómez-Martinez, S., & González-Soltero, R. (2022). *The influence of dietary factors on the gut microbiota.* Microorganisms, 10(7), 1368. https://doi.org/10.3390/microorganisms10071368

O'Connor, A. (2021, August 13). *How fermented foods may alter your microbiome and improve your health.* The New York Times. https://www.nytimes.com/2021/08/13/well/eat/yogurt-kimchi-kombucha-microbiome.html

O'Connor, B. (2016, August 19). *12 inspiring quotes about becoming vegetarian.* Doyou. https://www.doyou.com/12-inspiring-quotes-about-becoming-vegetarian-38264/

Ordovas, J. M., Ferguson, L. R., Tai, E. S., & Mathers, J. C. (2018). *Personalised nutrition and health.* BMJ, 361, bmj.k2173. https://doi.org/10.1136/bmj.k2173

Osamu, S. (2020, May). *The fermented foods of Tohoku.* GOVERNMENT of JAPAN. https://www.gov-online.go.jp/eng/publicity/book/hlj/html/202005/202005_05_en.html#:~:text=In%20Japan%20too%2C%20many%20types

Overview of the digestive system - Anatomy and Physiology. (n.d.). Openstax. https://openstax.org/books/anatomy-and-physiology/pages/23-1-overview-of-the-digestive-system

Panoff, L. (2021, February 12). *Sea moss: Benefits, nutrition, and preparation.* healthline. https://www.healthline.com/nutrition/seamoss

Parente, E. B., Harjutsalo, V., Lehto, M., Forsblom, C., Sandholm, N., & Groop, P.-H. (2020). *Relationship between ABO blood groups and cardiovascular disease in type 1 diabetes according to diabetic nephropathy status.* Cardiovascular Diabetology, 19(1). https://doi.org/10.1186/s12933-020-01038-z

Patrick Stump quote. (n.d.). Quotefancy. https://quotefancy.com/quote/1595760/Patrick-Stump-I-definitely-love-kimchi-The-biggest-influence-that-eating-so-much-Korean

Precision nutrition. (2020, September 23). Harvard SCHOOL of PUBLIC HEALTH. https://www.hsph.harvard.edu/nutritionsource/precision-nutrition/

Proietto, J. (2015, September 25). *Chemical messengers: How hormones make us feel hungry and full.* THE CONVERSATION. https://theconversation.com/chemical-messengers-how-hormones-make-us-feel-hungry-and-full-35545

Pullen, C. (2023, April 27). *13 Greek foods that are super healthy.* Healthline. https://www.healthline.com/nutrition/13-healthy-greek-foods

Purohit, M. (2015, June 5). *The effects of vegetarian diets on digestive health.* DoveMed. https://www.dovemed.com/healthy-living/wellness-center/effects-vegetarian-diets-digestive-health/

Quotes: Culture and food. (n.d.). FoodReference. https://www.foodreference.com/html/qculture.html

Red meat, processed meat and cancer. (n.d.). Cancer Council NSW. https://www.cancercouncil.com.au/1in3cancers/lifestyle-choices-and-cancer/red-meat-processed-meat-and-cancer/#:~:text=The%20World%20Health%20Organization%20has

Reddy, G., & van Dam, R. M. (2020). *Food, culture, and identity in multicultural societies: Insights from Singapore.* Appetite, 149, 104633. https://doi.org/10.1016/j.appet.2020.104633

Reis, A. (2022, May 26). *Nydelig! 27 popular Norwegian meal ideas.* Cooking Chew. https://cookingchew.com/norwegian-recipes.html

Rejeski, J. J., Wilson, F. M., Nagpal, R., Yadav, H., & Weinberg, R. B. (2021). *The impact of a Mediterranean diet on the gut microbiome in healthy human subjects: A pilot study.* Digestion, 1–8. https://doi.org/10.1159/000519445

Reynolds, S. (2018, October 1). *Gut communicates directly with brain.* National Institutes of Health (NIH). https://www.nih.gov/news-events/nih-research-matters/gut-communicates-directly-brain

Riaz Rajoka, M. S., Shi, J., Mehwish, H. M., Zhu, J., Li, Q., Shao, D., Huang, Q., & Yang, H. (2017). *Interaction between diet composition and gut microbiota and its impact on gastrointestinal tract health.* Food Science and Human Wellness, 6(3), 121–130. https://doi.org/10.1016/j.fshw.2017.07.003

Robertson, R. (2016, November 18). *9 ways to improve your gut bacteria, based on science.* Healthline. https://www.healthline.com/nutrition/improve-gut-bacteria%23:~:text=Eating%2520a%2520diverse%2520diet%2520rich%2520in%2520whole%2520foods

Robino, A., Concas, M. P., Catamo, E., & Gasparini, P. (2019). *A brief review of genetic approaches to the study of food preferences: Current knowledge and future directions.* Nutrients, 11(8), 1735. https://doi.org/10.3390/nu11081735

Rodrigues, V. F., Elias-Oliveira, J., Pereira, Í. S., Pereira, J. A., Barbosa, S. C., Machado, M. S. G., & Carlos, D. (2022). *Akkermansia muciniphila and gut immune system: A good friendship that attenuates Inflammatory Bowel Disease, obesity, and diabetes.* Frontiers in Immunology, 13. https://doi.org/10.3389/fimmu.2022.934695

Safari, Z., & Gérard, P. (2019). *The links between the gut microbiome and non-alcoholic fatty liver disease (NAFLD).* Cellular and Molecular Life Sciences, 76(8), 1541–1558. https://doi.org/10.1007/s00018-019-03011-w

Sansone, A. E. (2022, March 25). *Yes, probiotic drinks can improve gut health—We asked the experts which ones are best.* Prevention. https://www.prevention.com/food-nutrition/g39529307/best-probiotic-drinks/

Schnorr, S. L., & Bachner, H. A. (2016). *Integrative therapies in anxiety treatment with special emphasis on the gut microbiome.* The Yale Journal of Biology and Medicine, 89(3), 397–422. https://www.ncbi.nlm.nih.gov/pmc/articles/PMC5045149/

Serotonin: What is it, function & levels. (2022, March 18). Cleveland Clinic. https://my.clevelandclinic.org/health/articles/22572-serotonin

7 healthy Italian dishes that still taste amazing. (2019, December 30). De Nicolas Italian Dining. https://www.denicolasitaliandining.com/blog/7-healthy-italian-dishes-that-still-taste-amazing

Shiffer, E. (2023, May 15). *19 best foods for gut health.* Eat This Not That. https://www.eatthis.com/gut-healthy-foods/

Shmerling, R. H. (2017, May 12). *Diet not working? Maybe it's not your type.* Harvard Health Publishing. https://www.health.harvard.edu/blog/diet-not-working-maybe-its-not-your-type-2017051211678

Shoda, S. (2021). *Seeking prehistoric fermented food in Japan and Korea.* Current Anthropology, S000-S000. https://doi.org/10.1086/715808

Shubhangi. (2021, June 7). *10 famous healthy Indian foods and their calories.* Wellcurve. https://www.wellcurve.in/blog/famous-healthy-indian-foods/

Shubrook, N. (2019). *The health benefits of kimchi.* BBC Goodfood. https://www.bbcgoodfood.com/howto/guide/health-benefits-kimchi

Sibal, V. (2018, September). *Food: Identity of culture and religion.* ResearchGate. https://www.researchgate.net/publication/327621871_FOOD_IDENTITY_OF_CULTURE_AND_RELIGION

Singh, R. K., Chang, H.-W., Yan, D., Lee, K. M., Ucmak, D., Wong, K., Abrouk, M., Farahnik, B., Nakamura, M., Zhu, T. H., Bhutani, T., & Liao, W. (2017). *Influence of diet on the gut microbiome and implications for human health.* Journal of Translational Medicine, 15(1). https://doi.org/10.1186/s12967-017-1175-y

Sonnenburg, E. D., & Sonnenburg, J. L. (2019). *The ancestral and industrialized gut microbiota and implications for human health.* Nature Reviews Microbiology, 17(6), 383–390. https://doi.org/10.1038/s41579-019-0191-8

Spector, T. (2019, May 17). *15 tips to boost your gut microbiome.* BBC Science Focus Magazine. https://www.sciencefocus.com/the-human-body/how-to-boost-your-microbiome/

Stomach: Anatomy, function, diagram, parts of, structure. (2021, October 9). Cleveland Clinic. https://my.clevelandclinic.org/health/body/21758-stomach

Stoody, E., Obaggy, J., Pannucci, R., Fu, S., Rahavi, E., Altman, J., Adler, M., Brown, C., Scanlon, K., de Jesus, J., Olson, R., Perinne, C., Quam, J., Piercy, K., Vargas, A., Lerman, J., DeSilva, D., & Anderson-Villaluz, D. (2020). *Dietary guidelines for Americans 2020 -2025.* In Dietary Guidelines for Americans. https://www.dietaryguidelines.gov/sites/default/files/2020-12/Dietary_Guidelines_for_Americans_2020-2025.pdf

Sustainable eating is cheaper and healthier. (2021, November 11). University of Oxford. https://www.ox.ac.uk/news/2021-11-11-sustainable-eating-cheaper-and-healthier-oxford-study

Tamale. (2019, October 8). Wikipedia. https://en.wikipedia.org/wiki/Tamale

Tamang, J. P. (2014). *Fermented food - an overview.* ScienceDirect. https://www.sciencedirect.com/topics/agricultural-and-biological-sciences/fermented-food

Terry, S. M., Barnett, J. A., & Gibson, D. L. (2022). *A critical analysis of eating disorders and the gut microbiome.* Journal of Eating Disorders, 10(1). https://doi.org/10.1186/s40337-022-00681-z

The Associated Press. (2023, February 15). *A new study offers hints that healthier school lunches may help reduce obesity.* Npr. https://www.npr.org/2023/02/15/1157176728/healthy-school-meals-nutrition-obesity-study

The brain-gut connection. (2019). JOHN HOPKINS MEDICINE. https://www.hopkinsmedicine.org/health/wellness-and-prevention/the-brain-gut-connection

The digestive system and how it works. (2013). In National Institute of Diabetes and Digestive and Kidney Diseases. https://www.niddk.nih.gov/-/media/Files/Digestive-Diseases/Digestive_System_508.pdf

The gut-brain connection. (2019, April 19). Harvard Health Publishing. https://www.health.harvard.edu/diseases-and-conditions/the-gut-brain-connection

The mind-gut connection quotes by Emeran Mayer. (n.d.). Goodreads. https://www.goodreads.com/work/quotes/44319543-the-mind-gut-connection-how-the-astonishing-dialogue-taking-place-in-ou#:~:text=%E2%80%9CMany%20of%20the%20gut%20signals

The right plant-based diet for you. (2018). Harvard Health. https://www.health.harvard.edu/staying-healthy/the-right-plant-based-diet-for-you

Tomova, A., Bukovsky, I., Rembert, E., Yonas, W., Alwarith, J., Barnard, N. D., & Kahleova, H. (2019). *The effects of vegetarian and vegan diets on gut microbiota.* Frontiers in Nutrition, 6(47). https://doi.org/10.3389/fnut.2019.00047

Top 10 Cat Stevens quotes. (n.d.). BrainyQuote. https://www.brainyquote.com/lists/authors/top-10-cat-stevens-quotes#:~:text=I%20became%20a%20vegetarian%2C%20and,special%20drinks%20everywhere%20I%20went.&text=A%20person%20who%20steals%20bread,not%20treated%20as%20a%20thief.

Top 10 fermented foods for great gut health. (2022, December 30). Happy Kombucha. https://happykombucha.co.uk/blogs/happykombucha-1/top-10-fermented-foods-for-great-gut-health

Top 25 American diet quotes. (n.d.). AZ QUOTES. https://www.azquotes.com/quotes/topics/american-diet.html

Top 25 plant-based diet quotes. (n.d.). AZ QUOTES. https://www.azquotes.com/quotes/topics/plant-based-diet.html

Torrens, K. (2023, March 24). *Top 5 health benefits of sea moss.* Goodfood; BBC Good Food. https://www.bbcgoodfood.com/howto/guide/top-5-health-benefits-of-sea-moss

25 healthy eating quotes to motivate you to make better choices. (2021, January 19). Yahoo! https://www.yahoo.com/lifestyle/9-healthy-eating-quotes-motivate-150000510.html

Tzameli, I. (n.d.). *Special issue: Neuroendocrine control of appetite.* In Cell PRESS. https://www.cell.com/trends/endocrinology-metabolism/pdf/S1043-2760(12)00220-2.pdf

UNESCO - Washoku, traditional dietary cultures of the Japanese, notably for the celebration of New Year. (n.d.). Unesco. https://ich.unesco.org/en/RL/washoku-traditional-dietary-cultures-of-the-japanese-notably-for-the-celebration-of-new-year-00869#:~:text=Washoku%20is%20a%20social%20practice

van de Wouw, M., Boehme, M., Lyte, J. M., Wiley, N., Strain, C., O'Sullivan, O., Clarke, G., Stanton, C., Dinan, T. G., & Cryan, J. F. (2018). *Short-chain fatty acids: microbial metabolites that alleviate stress-induced brain-gut axis alterations.* The Journal of Physiology, 596(20), 4923–4944. https://doi.org/10.1113/jp276431

Variety is the spice of life | Phrase definition, origin & examples. (n.d.). GINGER. https://www.gingersoftware.com/content/phrases/variety-is-the-spice-of-life/

Vijay, A., & Valdes, A. M. (2021). *Role of the gut microbiome in chronic diseases: a narrative review.* European Journal of Clinical Nutrition, 1–13. https://doi.org/10.1038/s41430-021-00991-6

Virani, S. S., Alonso, A., Benjamin, E. J., Bittencourt, M. S., Callaway, C. W., Carson, A. P., Chamberlain, A. M., Chang, A. R., Cheng, S., Delling, F. N., Djousse, L., Elkind, M. S. V., Ferguson, J. F., Fornage, M., Khan, S. S., Kissela, B. M., Knutson, K. L., Kwan, T. W., Lackland, D. T., & Lewis, T. T. (2020). *Heart disease and stroke statistics—2020 update.* Circulation, 141(9). https://doi.org/10.1161/cir.0000000000000757

Waite, R. (2018). *2018 will see high meat consumption in the U.S., but the American diet is shifting.* WORLD RESOURCES INSTITUTE. https://www.wri.org/insights/2018-will-see-high-meat-consumption-us-american-diet-shifting

Wang, Y., & Beydoun, M. A. (2009). *Meat consumption is associated with obesity and central obesity among US adults.* International Journal of Obesity, 33(6), 621–628. https://doi.org/10.1038/ijo.2009.45

Wang, Y., Uffelman, C. N., Bergia, R. E., Clark, C. M., Reed, J. B., Cross, T.-W. L., Lindemann, S. R., Tang, M., & Campbell, W. W. (2022). *Meat consumption and gut microbiota: A scoping review of literature and systematic review of randomized controlled trials in adults.* Advances in Nutrition. https://doi.org/10.1016/j.advnut.2022.10.005

Watson, S. (2013, December 11). *The blood type diet.* WebMD. https://www.webmd.com/diet/a-z/blood-type-diet

Weaver, J. (2021, July 12). *A fermented-food diet increases microbiome diversity and lowers inflammation, Stanford study finds.* Standford Medicine. https://med.stanford.edu/news/all-news/2021/07/fermented-food-diet-increases-microbiome-diversity-lowers-inflammation

Wexler, J. (2020, February 14). *Climate impact of meat, vegetarian and vegan diets.* Ethical Consumer. https://www.ethicalconsumer.org/food-drink/climate-impact-meat-vegetarian-vegan-diets

What are the benefits of sea moss? (2021, December 22). Cleveland Clinic. https://health.clevelandclinic.org/sea-moss-benefits/

What are the best sources of protein? (2021, July 7). Cleveland Clinic. https://health.clevelandclinic.org/what-are-the-best-sources-of-protein/

What should I eat for a healthy gut? (2019, August 27). BBC FOOD. https://www.bbc.co.uk/food/articles/what_should_you_eat_for_a_healthy_gut

Whole grains with a Mediterranean flair. (2022, January 5). The Whole Grains Council. https://wholegrainscouncil.org/blog/2022/01/whole-grains-mediterranean-flair#:~:text=a%20big%20way.-

Widmer, R. J., Flammer, A. J., Lerman, L. O., & Lerman, A. (2015). *The Mediterranean diet, its components, and cardiovascular disease.* The American Journal of Medicine, 128(3), 229–238. https://doi.org/10.1016/j.amjmed.2014.10.014

Wolff, A. (2008, July 9). *Soul food.* Encyclopedia Britannica. https://www.britannica.com/topic/soul-food-cuisine

Wong, C. (2014, August 20). *What is the blood type fit?* Verywellfit. https://www.verywellfit.com/the-blood-type-diet-89893

Wu, Y., Wan, J., Choe, U., Pham, Q., Schoene, N. W., He, Q., Li, B., Yu, L., & Wang, T. T. Y. (2019). *Interactions between food and gut microbiota: Impact on human health.* Annual Review of Food Science and Technology, 10(1), 389–408. https://doi.org/10.1146/annurev-food-032818-121303

Your digestive system & how it works. (2023, May 11). National Institute of Diabetes and Digestive and Kidney Diseases. https://www.niddk.nih.gov/health-information/digestive-diseases/digestive-system-how-it-works

Zakira Naureen, Bonetti, G., Maria Chiara Medori, Aquilanti, B., Velluti, V., Matera, G., Iaconelli, A., & Bertelli, M. (2022). *Foods of the Mediterranean diet: lacto-fermented food, the food pyramid and food combinations.* 63(2 Suppl 3), E28–E35. https://doi.org/10.15167/2421-4248/jpmh2022.63.2s3.2744

Zhu, F., Tu, H., & Chen, T. (2022). *The microbiota–gut–brain axis in depression: The potential pathophysiological mechanisms and microbiota combined antidepression effect.* Nutrients, 14(10), 2081. https://doi.org/10.3390/nu14102081

Made in United States
Troutdale, OR
11/03/2026

56845383R00106